Community Based Nursing Curriculum:
A Faculty Guide

If you've enjoyed *Community-based Nursing: A Faculty Guide*, take a look at its companion undergraduate textbook —*Community-based Nursing Practice: Learning Through Students' Stories*—and see what it can do for your students. In the textbook, the authors of *A Faculty Guide* prepare students for meaningful clinical experiences in community-based settings.

Sorrell and Redmond teach students how to employ skills they have already mastered in their fundamentals classes in different community-based settings.

Here's what you will find in the student text:

- Engaging student stories incorporated throughout the text that make difficult concepts easy to understand

- Nursing as it really happens in community-based settings—with the chronically ill, families, and groups; in childcare centers, senior centers, elementary schools, college campuses, HIV/AIDS network, home care, and faith communities

- E-mail conversations between American and Canadian students that illustrate the commonalities and differences between community-based practice in the two countries

- Learning exercises in each chapter that emphasize active learning

- Clear differentiation between community-based practice and public health

- Coverage of alternative therapies and cultural and social issues

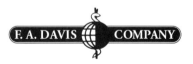

The Taber's Publisher

For additional information, contact F. A. Davis's customer service representatives at 800-323-3555 (US) or 800-665-1148 (Can) or e-mail us at orders@fadavis.com.

Community-based Nursing Curriculum:
A Faculty Guide

By

Georgine M. Redmond, RN, EdD

Associate Professor

College of Nursing and Health Science

George Mason University

Fairfax, Virginia

and

Jeanne M. Sorrell, RN, PhD

Professor

College of Nursing and Health Science

George Mason University

Fairfax, Virginia

F. A. Davis Company
1915 Arch Street
Philadelphia, PA 19103
www.fadavis.com

Copyright © 2002 by F. A. Davis Company

All rights reserved. This book is protected by copyright. No part of it may be reproduced, stored in a retrieval system, or transmitted in any form or by any means, electronic, mechanical, photocopying, recording, or otherwise, without written permission from the publisher.

Printed in the United States of America

Last digit indicates print number: 10 9 8 7 6 5 4 3 2 1

Acquisitions Editor: Joanne DaCunha
Developmental Editor: Ron Watson
Production Editor: Bette Haitsch
Designer: Melissa Walters
Cover Designer: Louis J. Forgione

As new scientific information becomes available through basic and clinical research, recommended treatments and drug therapies undergo changes. The author(s) and publisher have done everything possible to make this book accurate, up to date, and in accord with accepted standards at the time of publication. The authors, editors, and publisher are not responsible for errors or omissions or for consequences from application of the book, and make no warranty, expressed or implied, in regard to the contents of the book. Any practice described in this book should be applied by the reader in accordance with professional standards of care used in regard to the unique circumstances that may apply in each situation. The reader is advised always to check product information (package inserts) for changes and new information regarding dose and contraindications before administering any drug. Caution is especially urged when using new or infrequently ordered drugs.

Library of Congress Cataloging-in-Publication Data
Redmond, Georgine.
  Community-based nursing curriculum : a faculty guide / Georgine Redmond and Jeanne Sorrell. p. cm.
  Includes bibliographical references and index.
  ISBN 0-8036-0608-7
  1. Community health nursing. 2. Community health nursing—Study and teaching. 3. Nursing—Study and teaching. I. Sorrell, Jeanne Merkle. II. Title.

RT98 .R43 2002
610.73′43′071—dc21

2001042228

Authorization to photocopy items for internal or personal use, or the internal or personal use of specific clients, is granted by F. A. Davis Company for users registered with the Copyright Clearance Center (CCC) Transactional Reporting Service, provided that the fee of $.10 per copy is paid directly to CCC, 222 Rosewood Drive, Danvers, MA 01923. For those organizations that have been granted a photocopy license by CCC, a separate system of payment has been arranged. The fee code for users of the Transactional Reporting Service is: 8036-0608-7/02 0 + $.10.

DEDICATION

This book is dedicated to those who know, love, and have sustained us as we have developed this book:

The Lord, who is our "rock, fortress, and deliverer."

Our families:

Husband—Bob Redmond;
Children—Kelly, Kimberly, and Christopher;
Grandchildren—Brooke, Holly, and Emma.

Husband—Greg Sorrell; Children—Jeannette and Christine.

Dear friends and faculty colleagues.

—GR and JS

FOREWORD

The decade of the 1990s witnessed dramatic changes in health care in our country. In retrospect, Americans generally were fairly complacent about health care throughout the 1980s. All knew that our system offered the best there was to have—the best hospitals, the best nurses and doctors, the best specialty care, and the best technology that had been developed. Health care was a given—the full gamut of services were expected, even seen as an entitlement. But an undercurrent of concern about percentage of budget dollars spent, along with issues of cost, quality, and access were beginning to surface. You may remember a time before disease-related groups (DRGs).

In 1992, a new federal administration focused sharply on health care, and the American health-care bubble burst, bringing about spending caps, covered lives, limited stays, managed care, and a shift to care in the community. The community—what better place for nurses to take the lead? After all, isn't community care at the root of how nursing started? Yes and no.

Yes, nursing has had a strong presence in the community throughout its history and in this country; we all acknowledge the era of the Henry Street Settlement. But the "no" part of the equation relates to the change in the type of care given in the community. In this new community shift, nurses need not only to continue traditional community health roles and functions, but also to learn acute and primary care roles, skills, and responsibilities.

For those of us in nursing education, this new challenge raised imprtant questions. How should we respond? How should nursing education position itself? There was no paved path, and a major shift in curriculum was not something to be considered lightly.

In the College of Nursing and Health Science at George Mason University, it was clear that we needed to act quickly to do many things. Information had to be gained in regard to what was the actual situation—we needed a community assessment to identify the community needs. What were the acute and primary care skills needed? What types and kinds of placements and supervision did our students need? What were the curriculum changes that we needed to make? How were we going to handle this changing culture for both students and faculty? It is fair to say that both students and faculty had a tertiary-care philosophy, and students held expectations that their employment choices would be in critical care, EDs, and ICUs. Thinking about entry into practice in the community and not in the hospital was a major paradigm shift for both students and faculty. Many faculty needed and requested help through in-service workshops and colleague sharing. Performance outcomes had to be rethought and evaluation tools reworked or newly constructed.

In doing all these things and more, we learned what worked and what didn't. This book is geared to sharing that knowledge with colleagues who are at some stage in this curricular process, who want to know what other programs are doing, or who want guidelines and new ideas.

The faculty who have shared their expertise and stories in this book are all dedicated to a community-based curriculum, one that is timely, responsive, rich in knowledge and experience, and, most of all, prepares our graduates to function in the real world of health care as we know it today.

Rita M. Carty, RN, D.N.Sc., FAAN
Dean and Professor
George Mason University
Fairfax, Virginia

ACKNOWLEDGMENTS

The idea for this book grew out of our attempt to communicate to our professional colleagues how to develop and implement a community-based curriculum. Through consultation with other nursing programs, this volume began.

The contributions of faculty who teach the undergraduate nursing coursework are gratefully acknowledged. They alone weave the tapestry of knowledge and experience into a meaningful whole as we educate the nurses of tomorrow. Their dedication to students and student learning is exceptional.

Our dean, Rita M. Carty, is acknowledged for her support of this vision, and her encouragement to write what we "know" and "do."

Research assistants over the years of manuscript development are acknowledged for their many and varied contributions from literature reviews for authors to securing the myriad of permissions to publish the text: Shelley J. Kollar, Judith A. Rogers, Pamela R. Cangelosi, and Nancy L. Sloan.

We also wish to recognize the tireless efforts of administrative assistants: Louanne Pearce, early in the manuscript development, and Nasim Khawaja, who has sustained this effort. Laura Sykes, our photographer, also participated in several marathon days to get the best pictures for our text.

The F.A. Davis staff is also acknowledged, particularly Joanne P. DaCunha, for her creativity and enthusiasm.

Acknowledgments for Student Stories

We would like to acknowledge the following students, including those who wish to remain anonymous, for their contributions

Students from George Mason University

- Mary Afshar
- Madonna C. Arellano
- Eric Cohen
- Ruth Dimaranan
- Lynn Grillo
- Michael E. Iduma
- Diana M. Jones
- Rita Kathalynas
- Ann Marie Limner
- Paige R. Migliozzi
- Kathryn F. Rau

CONTRIBUTORS

Christine T. Blasser, RN, MSN
Instructor
College of Nursing and Health Science
George Mason University
Fairfax, Virginia

M. Lucille Boland, RN, MSN
Assistant Professor
College of Nursing and Health Science
George Mason University
Fairfax, Virginia

Susan W. Durham, RN, MPH
Instructor
College of Nursing and Health Science
George Mason University
Fairfax, Virginia

Carol J. Huddleston, RN, MN
Clinical Instructor
College of Nursing and Health Science
George Mason University
Fairfax, Virginia

Joanne C. Langan, RN, PhD
Adjunct Assistant Professor
School of Nursing
St. Louis University
St. Louis, Missouri

Christena Langley, RN, PhD
Assistant Professor, Clinical Management Coordinator
College of Nursing and Health Science
George Mason University
Fairfax, Virginia

Margaret A. Miklancie, RN, PhD
Former Coordinator, Undergraduate Nursing Program, Upper Division
College of Nursing and Health Science
George Mason University
Fairfax, Virginia

Margaret M. Moss, RN, MSN
Instructor
College of Nursing and Health Science
George Mason University
Fairfax, Virginia

Loretta Brush Normile, RN, PhD
Assistant Professor
College of Nursing and Health Science
George Mason University
Fairfax, Virginia

Georgine M. Redmond, RN, EdD
Former Associate Dean, Undergraduate Programs
Associate Professor
College of Nursing and Health Science
George Mason University
Fairfax, Virginia

Jeanne M. Sorrell, RN, PhD
Coordinator, Professor, PhD Program in Nursing
College of Nursing and Health Science
George Mason University
Fairfax, Virginia

REVIEWERS

Ida Androwich, RN, PhD, FAAN
Associate Professor
Loyola University of Chicago
Maywood, Illinois

Carol Alvates Brooks, RN, DNSc
Associate Professor
Syracuse University
Syracuse, New York

Patricia A. Gonser, RN, PhD
Associate Professor
University of Southern Mississippi
Meridian, Mississippi

Rosemary Kohl, RN, MSN
Clinical Nurse Specialist, Medical Care Program,
BSN, and In-service Education
London Health Sciences Centre
London, Ontario, Canada

John R. Lowe, RN, PhD
Assistant Professor
Florida International University
Fort Lauderdale, Florida

M. Peggy MacLeod, RN, MN
Associate Professor
College of Nursing
University of Saskatchewan
Saskatoon, Saskatchewan

Sheila Favro Marks, RN, MS
Chair, Department of Nursing
Florida Southern College
Lakeland, Florida

Eleanor McClelland, RN, PhD, MPH
Associate Professor
The University of Iowa
College of Nursing
Iowa City, Iowa

Nancy J. Michela, RN,C, MS
Associate Professor
Russell Sage College
Troy, New York

Anne K. Moshtael, RN, BSN
Nursing Instructor
Macon Technical Institute
Macon, Georgia

Linda Pearce, RN,C, MEd, CDE, CPNA
Consultant
Clinical Practice
Brandon, Mississippi

Patricia Schafer, RN, PhD
Associate Professor
Carlow College
Pittsburgh, Pennsylvania

Julie A. Slack, RN, MSN(c)
Instructor of Nursing
Dixie College
St. George, Utah

Patricia Torsella, RN, DNSc
Associate Professor
Bloomsburg University
Bloomsburg, Pennsylvania

Carol Zeller, RN, MSN
Nursing Instructor
College of Marin
Kentfield, California

Contents

Section 1
General Concepts for Faculty in Community-based Sites

Chapter 1
>   Choosing and Contracting for Community-based Sites   3
>   Joanne C. Langan

Chapter 2
>   Selection of Faculty for a Community-based Curriculum   17
>   Margaret A. Miklancie

Chapter 3
>   Teaching through Stories: An Approach to Student-centered Learning   29
>   Jeanne M. Sorrell

Chapter 4
>   Teaching and Learning Activities in Community-based Settings   41
>   Georgine M. Redmond

Chapter 5
>   Preparing Students for Home Visits   53
>   Christine T. Blasser

Chapter 6
>   Teaching Students in Unstructured Community Settings   71
>   Christena Langley

Section 2

Faculty Application in Community-based Sites

Chapter 7
    Teaching Students in a Senior Center   95
    Joanne C. Langan

Chapter 8
    Teaching Students the Care of Underserved Children in an Elementary School   109
    Carol J. Huddleston

Chapter 9
    Teaching Students in a Campus Clinical   121
    M. Lucille Boland

Chapter 10
    Teaching Students in a Community HIV/AIDS Network   139
    Loretta Brush Normile

Chapter 11
    Teaching Students in a Home-care Setting   149
    Susan W. Durham

Chapter 12
    Teaching Students in a Faith Community   161
    Margaret M. Moss

Index   **179**

SECTION 1

General Concepts for Faculty in Community-based Sites

CHAPTER 1

Choosing and Contracting for Community-based Sites

Joanne C. Langan

Learning Objectives

1) Discuss the approaches to securing community-based sites.
2) Specify the advantages and disadvantages of "split" sites.
3) Describe the steps taken to secure a community-based contract with an agency.
4) Identify the key aspects of contracts that must be reviewed between the school and the agency.
5) Develop a list of potential community-based sites.

Schools of nursing have made major curriculum changes to meet the demand for nurses prepared to deliver health care in a variety of settings. Student clinical experiences take place in home and community settings because of the transfer of nursing care provision from acute care to the community (Noble et al. 1996). This chapter presents a background of the provision of community-based experiences, the importance of community partnerships, the steps in choosing and contracting for community-based sites, and, finally, my own story of obtaining contracts at George Mason University (GMU), College of Nursing and Health Science.

Community experiences provide the opportunity for students to learn patient care that they may never see within an institution. Outside of the traditional health-care settings, the students may see nurses practicing with greater autonomy in a variety of roles. Community clinicals also provide students with opportunities to explore their practice values and ethical decision making. De La Garza and Martinez-Rogers (1998) assert that students in community settings face issues such as conflict between "what is valued" and "what is," time allocation, access to care, scarce resources, and different cultural responses to illness.

Although they provide care in often less-than-desirable circumstances, the nursing students learn to be adaptable and flexible. The exposure to a wide variety of clients in a number of different living situations helps the students develop a more holistic view of nursing (Yoder et al. 1997). In this way, graduating students have a more realistic view of the emerging health-care delivery system in which they will practice (De La Garza & Martinez-Rogers 1998).

Note that experts in the fields of community health and public health make distinctions between community-based nursing and community health nursing. Zotti and colleagues (1996) define *community-based nursing* (CBN) as:

> a philosophy of nursing that guides nursing care provided for individuals, families, and groups wherever they are, including where they live, work, play, or go to school. CBN is characterized by an individual and family-centered orientation, the development of partnerships with clients, and an appreciation of the values of the community (p 211).

In contrast, *community health nursing* (CHN) is synonymous with "public health nursing." Zotti and colleagues (1996) define CHN by incorporating writings from the Public Health Nurse Section of the American Public Health Association, 1980 and 1996, and the Council of Community Health Nurses of the American Nurses Association:

> CHN represents a systematic process of delivering nursing care to improve the health of an entire community. Although CHN may deliver care to individuals and groups, it is primarily responsible for the health of the population as a whole, with special emphasis on identification of high-risk aggregates. CHN practice synthesizes nursing theory and public health science and places priority on prevention, protection, and promotion (p 212).

The distinction offered by these authors matches the differences between the community-focused clinicals that we at GMU offer our nursing students. The junior year of our baccalaureate program community clinical emphasizes work with individuals, families, and small groups, what Zotti and colleagues label "community-based nursing." Our senior nursing students focus on populations as a whole, with identification of high-risk aggregates, more in fitting with Zotti and colleague's definition of community health nursing.

At GMU's College of Nursing and Health Science, the goal of providing community-based nursing experiences is to assist the students in mastering assessment skills for providing collaborative nursing care to individuals, families, and small groups. An emphasis is placed on culturally diverse and vulnerable populations experiencing physiological, psychological, and social health problems in a variety of settings throughout the life span. Clients are viewed in their homes, where they work, and in the communities in which they live. The model used at GMU parallels a practicum for baccalaureate nursing students in a Department of Veterans Affairs home-care program as described by Gray and colleagues (1998). The model of Gray and coworkers includes direct patient care, support to caregivers, assessment, and referrals to community resources. Students in the VA model also conduct teaching projects to targeted populations. Clinical placements are sought in elementary schools, church communities, shelters, sheltered workshops, clinics, day care centers, health centers, and senior centers.

COMMUNITY PARTNERSHIPS

In each of these settings, we develop valued community partnerships. Partnership is defined in *Webster's New Basic Dictionary* (1997) as "a relationship resembling a legal partnership and usually involving close cooperation between parties having been specified and joint rights and responsibilities" (p 123). In fact, our partnerships are legal agreements between GMU's College of Nursing and Health Science and the community agency. In the legal agreements, also called *contracts* or *affiliation agreements,* the joint rights and responsibilities of both parties are defined. The close cooperation between parties is an integral element in the success of the shared endeavor. We at the College of Nursing and Health Science cannot fulfill our commitment to quality clinical experiences for our students without the express consent and cooperation of our community partners.

Yoder and colleagues (1997) shared the experience of their agency-university partnership. One of their strategies in developing a new community-based course was to hold a joint meeting with the course instructor, agency education coordinator, and preceptors to review course content and learning objectives. Yoder and coworkers' success was based on realistic expectations and preceptors' ownership of the program—in other words, agency nurses participated in the planning process. Another reason given for the success of the partnership was that written guidelines outlining the responsibilities of all parties were posted and used as a reference.

We must listen to our community experts regarding the types of skills and the level of expertise they desire in our new graduates. In turn, they must listen to the types of experiences the college is providing, make recommendations, and provide access to their agencies to improve the student preparation for practice. Hopefully, our nursing students and faculty members bring a richness to the agencies by providing needed teaching, faculty practice expertise, attention to clients, assessments and screenings, location of resources, services, and individual and family visits.

It may take some time for the clinical faculty and students to gain the trust of the clinical agencies and to "prove their value-added" ability, as one clinical faculty member shared. However, once the initial adjustment period is past, many new ideas for activities and other agency involvement often emerge. More partnerships are forged, and symbiotic relationships are enjoyed. The initial partnership often controls the access to future agencies. For example, one must learn which agency or organization has the legal control of access to other affiliated agencies or organizations. The school of nursing has the onus of responsibility to determine who is responsible for access to agencies and to seek that party for negotiations. Claiming ignorance is no excuse for not following protocol.

Another type of partnership that develops is interdisciplinary. Community-based faculty and students likely will come in contact with case managers, physicians, and social workers. Much can be learned from these experts, especially in the process of coordination of care. Armentrout (1998) describes a collaborative climate among health-care providers and various agencies in the community. She states that this cooperation fosters change, improves client care, and restores a sense of stability, yet enhances creativity. Zotti and colleagues (1996) suggest that students need opportunities to work in teams during clinical courses to enhance their abilities to understand their roles as team members.

Although much initial, informal dialogue occurs among our nursing administrators, faculty, and agency administrators, choices must be made among potential

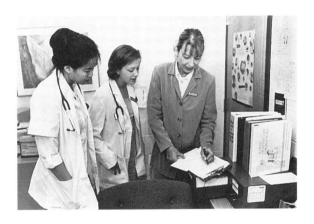

sites. Then, the first formal step in designing the community-based clinical experience is the negotiation of the contract.

There are many factors to consider when choosing and contracting for community-based sites. The needs and desires of the clinical agency as well as the nursing school and students are reviewed. This chapter discusses those key factors. Preliminary and extended reviews of all key factors make a successful learning experience and more likely pleased community clients.

Assessment

It is essential that the course objectives are clear when community-based sites are considered. The objectives must be measurable and definable. For instance, one must be able to list learning activities for each objective in which students will engage to achieve the objectives. More than one activity should be considered for each objective because the community-based sites vary so greatly. More than one means to achieve objectives may be necessary.

Student learning needs are reviewed for classes as a whole as well as for individuals. A basic assessment of individual students can be achieved by asking students to list previous clinical experiences and health care–related jobs, volunteer work, and life experiences. Generic or traditional student learning needs may vary greatly with registered nurse student learning needs. Some students may benefit from a reinforcement of concepts previously learned with individuals and families, whereas others may need exposure to new material and experiences in novel sites.

Securing Community-based Sites

Although finding and securing community-based sites can be a daunting task, there are ways to achieve the desired number of sites in the least painful manner. Some of the approaches to securing community-based sites include (1) reviewing contracts already in place, (2) eliciting faculty recommendations, (3) eliciting student recommendations, (4) considering agency invitations of faculty and students, and (5) community networking. The following discussion will explain each of these approaches.

Some contracts may have been secured for a specific clinical rotation, and the agency may be able to offer opportunities for broader student learning. For example, one agency may house long-term care clients, assisted living clients, and adult day care clients. The long-term care experience may be appropriate for learning basic nursing care in a beginning-level course, whereas the adult day care clients may provide community learning experiences focused on individuals and families. Perhaps the contract was secured for the initial long-term care experience, but it will still be valid with the agency for the community-based experience. Each agency should be considered for a broader base of opportunities than originally planned.

If faculty and students are made aware of the clinical site needs of the nursing program, they can assist with the generation of ideas for clinical placements. Again, faculty members may be using a site for a specific course and would be able to recommend that site for another clinical course if the site were utilized differently. Students often bring a tapestry of work and volunteer experiences with them to the nursing program. A senior nursing student recommended a site where she worked as a part-time receptionist. Because she was familiar with the curriculum, she recognized the potential of the site. Eventually, the site was "processed," and a contract was secured.

At times, an agency will call the nursing programs to ask for student involvement with the agency's clients. These contacts can result in mutually beneficial relationships between the agency and the nursing program.

Finally, all nursing faculty need to be ambassadors for the nursing program, facilitating the development of community-based sites through community networking. Community partnerships develop through networking with businesses, professional organizations, small groups, and committees. Many times, community-based sites are appropriate placements for both undergraduate and graduate students. An open mind is necessary to consider all possibilities.

The mini-exercise in Box 1–1 will help the reader in brainstorming potential clinical sites.

Box 1-1   Learning Exercise for Faculty Use

Developing and Creating Community-based Sites

List at least three agencies that you currently use as clinical sites that could be expanded to community-based sites.

List at least three agencies that you would consider using to achieve community-based curriculum objectives.

CONTACTING POTENTIAL AGENCIES

Initially, the clinical placement coordinator may contact the potential community-based site or agency director by phone. The purpose of the call is to describe how the placement coordinator perceives a potentially mutually beneficial relationship between the school and the agency. The agency must be informed of the level of student suggested for the agency, the number of students to be placed, and the length of time of the assignments (number of weeks, days of the week, hours per day). Whether the agency contacted the school or vice versa, a site visit should be requested so that the plant can be viewed and assessed first-hand by the placement coordinator.

Sharing Course Syllabi and Objectives with Agency

Sharing the course syllabus with potential clinical site directors gives the directors the opportunity to review course objectives and the overall expectations for student placement. The agency administrator may wish to review the syllabus prior to the placement coordinator's visit or choose to review it at the time of the initial visit.

Whether the agency administrator has the syllabus well in advance of the initial visit or is seeing the syllabus for the first time at the visit, each objective must be reviewed and discussed. In this way, both administrators can discuss how the objectives can be met or not met at the agency.

In addition to assessing the agency's ability to assist students in meeting course objectives, the number of students that can be accommodated at the site must be discussed. For example, if a clinical section has 10 students, one needs to know if there is physical space for all to gather with the faculty member. If students are to do individual and family assessments, one needs to be assured that 10 individual families will be accessible to the students.

If all 10 students cannot be accommodated at one site, the clinical section may be divided between two sites. The two sites should be in close geographical proximity and be complementary to one another. For example, a residential institution for mentally retarded adults was used as a site for five students, and the other five students were placed at a hospital's child care and development center. At mid-semester, the students traded places. The students compared and contrasted clients' developmental levels and parents' perceptions of the health of their children at both sites. Parents of children at the child care center were more accessible than parents of the residential clients. In this circumstance, modifications in meeting course objectives may need to be made based on individual, family, group, and agency differences.

If it is anticipated that students may be split between two clinical sites, consider the following advantages and disadvantages of split sites.

Advantages of Split Sites

- Exposure to two very different kinds of agencies, clients, and their families
- A better understanding of the variability in the definition of "family"
- An opportunity to observe a collaborative, interdisciplinary approach to the care of residential clients in specialized weekly clinics (for instance, orthopedic clinic)
- An opportunity to see nurses function as care coordinators for distinctly different disorders
- An opportunity to learn proper feeding methods for infants, children, and those with feeding tubes or motor disabilities
- An opportunity to observe and initiate creative ways of administering medications to children and disabled individuals

Disadvantages of Split Sites

- Faculty members must divide their time between sites.
- Time that should be spent with students is lost as the faculty members travel between sites.
- Faculty members must decide how to divide their time between sites such as alternate days at sites or split days between the two sites.
- Personnel at the agency must be comfortable with the lack of constant faculty supervision; there must be a preceptor identified for the students to contact in the faculty member's absence.

- A registered nurse is not always available at each site to model nurse behaviors to students, so that faculty members become the models and are not always present.
- Students may not feel that they had enough time to develop therapeutic relationships with the individual clients and their families when they must switch sites midway through the semester.

When all of these issues are considered, weigh the benefits and risks to the choice of split sites. Working in more than one community-based site many enrich the students' experience, but some compromise and additional effort will be needed by the faculty member.

> **Box 1-2** Learning Exercise for Faculty Use
>
> ### Student Placement
>
> You are a faculty member in Amos University's community-based nursing program. In the second semester of the junior year, students are assigned to community-based sites to work with individuals, groups, and families. One instructor is assigned to each group of 10 students. Some instructors are split with their students among two to three agencies. Others are on-site with their clinical students in one agency.
>
> You are making student placement decisions. Make a list of the characteristics of the student you would assign to a split site. Give your rationale.

In addition to the faculty member's willingness to "go the extra mile" and participate actively in teaching students, clients, and often, agency personnel, the ability of the students to provide support to the agency is another benefit to the agencies.

SERVICE LEARNING

Service learning has been discussed as students serving the community by applying what they learn in their courses and curriculum to help improve the lives of people living in their communities (Greenberg 1999). Service learning is also the process of integrating community service and critical-thinking exercises into the curriculum to enhance and enrich student learning and development. *Experiential learning* is the philosophical foundation of service learning. Service learning directly engages the student in the subject matter being studied to enrich the learning experience. The emphasis is on both student learning and benefit to the community. Service learning activities include those that address the human, safety, educational, and environmental needs of the community (Gaither et al 1998).

The concept of service learning is an important selling point to agencies when negotiating for access to the agency with the hope of securing a contract. Agencies need to understand that the students are capable of providing services to individuals and the community through the opportunity of a partnership with the agency. Potential community partners want to hear about what the students have learned in the classroom about their particular clients and how they have been prepared to be of assistance to the community.

The didactic courses in community-based nursing are taken concurrently with the clinical community course. In this way, the learner is well aware of the subject matter and key concepts involved in providing nursing care in community-based settings. Clinical learning experiences can be tailored to "fit" what has been learned in the classroom. For example, if safety considerations in the home are taught in the classroom, the students may look for these safety considerations in clients' homes or in the community setting where they work with clients.

While examining the clients' environment, the students may also make recommendations to improve the environment. Better ventilation, improved lighting, or removal of throw rugs or trip hazards may be suggested. Constant assessment and reassessment of the individuals, families, safety, and learning and environmental needs are made throughout the course of the semester. Students learn to develop their therapeutic communication techniques to elicit vital information as well as develop their critical-thinking skills as they assist clients with problem solving. By applying theory to practice in the community settings, the students learn by doing and benefit the individuals, families, small groups, and communities.

Mutually Beneficial Relationship

Whereas the nursing program administrator wants to contract with agencies that can meet course objectives, the agency administrator wants to know what the students and faculty member can do for the agency. The nursing program administrator may anticipate the following questions offered by Yoder and colleagues (1997): "How will students adjust and practice nursing in this complex setting? Are there benefits for (the) agency and the nurses? Can an experience be organized in such a way that it does not require an unrealistic investment of agency resources or decrease staff productivity?" (p 493). Student presence may not be perceived to be an asset but more an impediment to efficient daily agency operations (Yoder et al. 1997). To have a truly mutually beneficial relationship, there must be a clear description of expectations of the agency, the students, and faculty member.

It is important that the nursing program administrator approaches the negotiations armed with a list of activities and services that the students and faculty can do and provide. For instance, some of the community-based activities and services include those listed in Table 1–1.

Additionally, the agency may have some expectations for the students and faculty involving their participation in tasks that would benefit the agency. For example, the agency may request that the students present in-services for the agency staff, parents, or families. A list of some of these in-services is found in Table 1–2.

Table 1-1
Sample List of Activities and Services Students and Faculty Can Provide

Denver Developmental Screening Test (DDST)

Heights and Weights

Mini–Mental Status Exam

Vital Signs

Screenings: Vision, Hearing

Primary Care Teaching: Exercise
　　　　　　　　　　　　Healthy Eating
　　　　　　　　　　　　Stress Management
　　　　　　　　　　　　Explanation of Medicines

Poison Control

Table 1-2
Sample List of In-services

Proper hydration with the use of Metamucil

How to operate a Thermoscan

What blood pressure really measures

How to obtain an accurate blood pressure reading

Exercise tailored to the young or elderly

Therapeutic communication

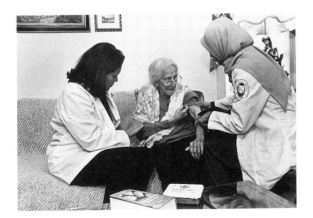

Specific teaching projects that nursing students may complete and present are also of interest to potential community-based sites. A sample list is found in Table 1–3.

There have been instances when agencies have asked students to perform more secretarial or menial tasks. Faculty members must be careful not to commit students to activities in which there is no learning value. However, simple tasks that may improve and facilitate positive relationships between agencies and the nursing program need to be considered for their merit before the faculty member quickly refuses their inclusion. An example of this situation happened to the author. We were asked to escort adult day-care clients to the agency's in-house beauty shop. At first glance, this may have seemed a task with no learning value, but it turned out to be a positive learning experience. Students reinforced their skill of transferring clients from chair to wheelchair, strengthened their knowledge of wheelchair safety, and took the opportunity to strengthen therapeutic communication techniques.

AFFILIATION AGREEMENTS

When it is decided that both the nursing program and the clinical agency will participate in a mutually beneficial relationship, the contract or affiliation agreement is reviewed. The nursing school typically initiates the contract, although the clinical agency has the option of using its contract, if one exists. Several key aspects of the contract must be reviewed. These key aspects include the legal terms, requirements of both parties, and the liability of both parties.

All legal terms must be clearly understood by all parties. The agency administrators will review the school's contract. Though these contracts or affiliation agreements may be standard for the school, they may appear strange or threatening to the clinical agency. The administrators need to understand that they are not obligated to accept students for clinical experiences every semester or even every year. Contracts are generally valid for a period of 3 years. Some schools have open-ended contracts that are valid until either party chooses to end the contract. However, some agencies prefer that contracts be reviewed and renewed annually. It is also important to advise the agency administrator to review the affiliation agreement with the agency's legal counsel so that all parties are comfortable with the language and requirements of the contract. Legal terms and contract language may require explanation by the nursing school

Table 1-3

Sample List of Nursing Student Teaching Projects

Practical tips on the use and care of hearing aids
Dental hygiene/tooth brushing
Dental hygiene/dentures
Hepatitis B
Safety in the home
Tracheostomy care
Preparing for diagnostic studies
Skin cancer/melanoma screening
Immunizations
Blood glucose monitoring
Breast self-exam
Good cholesterol/bad cholesterol
Playground rules and safety
Handwashing
How to keep your cold to yourself
Improving communications with Alzheimer's patients
Progressive phases of Alzheimer's disease
Facts about high blood pressure
Medications that should and should not be used by older adults
Questions to ask about residential care
Community resources for the elderly

administrator responsible for contracts or by the school's attorneys.

Both the nursing school program and the clinical agency need to clearly understand the legal liability and the expectations of each participating member. The contract will identify specific terms that are the legal responsibility of the clinical agency and those that are the legal responsibility of the nursing school program. For instance, the clinical agency retains ultimate responsibility for the clients in its care, while they are in its care. However, the students' and faculty members' actions are under the purview of the nursing school program. Each student and faculty member is responsible and accountable for his or her own actions, but the liability for their actions, if in error, is the legal responsibility of the nursing school. Students may be required to provide their own transportation, to attend mandatory orientation programs offered by the agency, and to wear agency identification badges.

As stated earlier, the nursing school program typically offers the standard contract to the clinical agency. In some cases, the agency may wish to use its contract or affiliation agreement or to change some of the language of the school's contract. The nursing school's administrator needs to consult with the school's legal department regarding the requested language changes. Although language changes do not typically cause major discrepancies, the legal department will need to determine that the changes maintain compliance with the contracting guidelines for the location or state of the school.

Finally, the nursing school administrator responsible for contracts must secure the signatures of the principal parties of both the school and agency. If the dean or director of the college or school of nursing has signature authority, she or he may sign for the school's interest. If this authority is not within the department, school, or college level, signatures must be sought from the appropriate person or persons. When all required signatures are secured, copies of the fully executed documents (contracts) are to be filed with both the nursing school and the community-based agency. In large schools or colleges that have many affiliation agreements, electronic files may be preferred over the storage of hard copies.

CONSULTATION WITH FACULTY MEMBER ASSIGNED TO AGENCY

After the relationship with the community-based site has been established and a contract secured, the nursing school's administrator has much to do to prepare the clinical faculty member for a successful experience in the agency. A thorough review of the affiliation agreement should be done with the faculty member. In this way, the faculty member becomes more cognizant of legal responsibilities and liabilities of the instructor and the clinical agency.

The clinical instructor assumes many roles in the clinical setting. The clinical instructor may be sought out by the agency as a health-care consultant and expert.

As teacher, the instructor guides the students toward achievement of course objectives and valuable applied learning experiences. As supervisor of students, the instructor is responsible for teaching the students responsibility and accountability for their actions as well as for supervising and being aware of those student actions. The instructor's close supervision clearly lessens the burden of oversight for the agency. As Yoder and coworkers (1997) caution, "It is highly critical that the instructor is directly involved and visible in the agency to help the students handle clinical and logistical problems that arise, such as a student becoming ill or having transportation problems. These strategies help to offset the view that the students are a 'bother'" (p 96). Again, the clinical agency retains ultimate responsibility for the clients; the faculty member is responsible for the students.

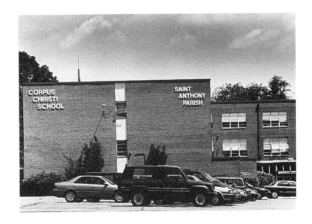

Clinical Supervision

It is strongly advised that the faculty member become familiar with policies of the agency and the nursing school. For example, it may be a school policy that all clinical faculty members wear a paging device so that they can be reached by students, nursing school, and agency personnel quickly. The beeper, however, does not diminish the supervisory role of the instructor; the instructor is expected to be visible and accessible to the students. This availability concept must be emphasized. The instructor is not free to take care of personal matters, business, or return to his or her home during the clinical day. Besides setting up a potentially disastrous situation, it is unethical to take care of personal matters while employed to supervise and teach students. To avoid the pitfalls of reliance on the personal pager, we developed a lengthy and specific list of supervisory guidelines for clinical faculty. Although some may consider the guidelines an insult to the professional nursing instructor, it is much better to outline and clarify expectations before the semester begins or untoward situations occur. Table 1–4 provides a sample of Guidelines for Clinical Supervision used in our college.

In the case of emergency or the faculty's inability to be present on a regularly scheduled clinical day, a plan should be in place for substitute clinical faculty or some other means of supervising the students in clinical. If there is no possibility of supervision of students in the clinical setting, provisions must be made to put a contingency plan in place. This plan should be on file in the college of nursing so that college administrators are able to access the plan in the faculty member's absence. The contingency plan activity choices need to address the clinical objectives for that day. The use and rationale of the contingency plan must be explained to the clinical agency as well as the means of contacting the agency regarding faculty member and student absence. A sample of a contingency plan that the author created is presented in Table 1–5.

The clinical agency may have specific policies regarding health-care persons and relationships with clients that the faculty member must be aware of and communicate to students. Other types of specific agency policies deal with emergency situations and proper transport of

Table 1-4

GMU's College of Nursing and Health Science Guidelines for Clinical Supervision in Community-based Sites

1. Clinical conferences will meet at least once a week with all students in attendance.
2. Students will be assigned a contact person in each agency. A BSN nurse, if available, is preferable. The function of the contact person is to provide direction and problem solving if the faculty member is not on-site.
3. Each clinical faculty member will provide the agencies with his or her schedule and beeper number. In addition, each faculty member will provide a weekly schedule. Students will also receive copies of the schedule.
4. Guidelines for clinical supervision should be provided to all course faculty by the course coordinator and discussed at the first course meeting.
5. Course objectives will be delivered to the agency and to preceptors each semester.
6. Clinical faculty will have contingency plans. Contingency plans are only to be used in an emergency. The definition of a contingency plan is an alternative plan in lieu of going to the clinical agency. Contingency plans and telephone trees should be developed by the end of the first week of class and submitted to the course coordinator and the associate dean for undergraduate programs.
7. Students may attend clinical activities on non-scheduled clinical days only if faculty supervision is available and if it is within the specifications of the agency contract.
8. Faculty in consultation with the course coordinator may assign seminars/conferences or other activities *only* if these are congruent with the objectives of the clinical course.
9. If multiple clinical sites are used for one clinical section, the faculty member will always be in one of those sites or enroute.
10. With all community clinical sections, including those for RNs, the faculty member will visit each clinical site at least once each semester.
11. All student clinical hours should be tracked. Clinical logs may be used for this purpose.

*A scheduled conference or meeting does not constitute an emergency and appropriate arrangements should be made for coverage.

> **Table 1-5**
>
> **GMU's College of Nursing and Health Science Contingency Plan—NURS 341, Section 210**
>
> 1. Students will scan the newspapers, current journals and magazines for health promotion, disease prevention articles for the senior population. Following a study of at least three varied sources, the student will compose a written report documenting:
>   A. The topic of each of the sources
>   B. Common themes of the articles
>   C. Differences among the articles
>   D. How the same medical/health care issues were addressed by each of the authors
>   E. The readability of each piece (i.e., would the target audience be able to understand and use the information easily?)
>
>   The written report will not exceed five typed pages, double-spaced, APA format. All sources must be cited.
>
> 2. Check the Medication Administration Records (MARs) from both Adult Day Care and Assisted Living areas of the Health Care Center. List all the medications prescribed for participants and residents (choose five persons).
>   A. Describe the most commonly prescribed medicines.
>   B. Study and describe the medicines' indications for use and side effects.
>   C. Answer: Are any of the medicines contraindicated for the same person?
>   D. Answer: Are any of the medicines prescribed to counter side effects of other medicines?
>   E. Answer: Are the doses appropriate for the age of the clients? Weight?
>   F. Answer: What parameters are "vital" to assess before giving the medicines? (i.e., check apical pulse for 1 full min before administering digoxin)
>   G. Answer: Do you think the medicines prescribed for the individuals are appropriate? (i.e., do you see a match between the diagnoses and the medicines' indications?)
>   H. Answer: Do the individuals know what their medicines are and for what reason they are taking them?
>   I. Answer: What are the nursing actions/teaching points that are important for each medicine? What lab work should be monitored?
>   J. Answer: What would your nursing action be if you suspected one of your clients was experiencing an adverse effect of a medicine or combination of medicines?
>
>   Responses must be typed, double-spaced.
>
> ---
>
> *All contingency assignments are due to the instructor within 2 weeks of the missed clinical day, unless a written contract for an extension is submitted to the instructor and approved. The above contingency assignments address clinical objectives 1, 3, 4, 10.
>
> Source: Joanne C. Langan, George Mason University, College of Nursing and Health Science.

disabled clients. The proactive approach to knowledge about these policies is a much better public relations strategy than to find out about these policies following an unfortunate incident.

The author strongly encourages one to several instructor visits to the clinical agency in advance of the clinical start date. These visits allow the faculty member and clinical agency personnel to become familiar with each other. Expectations of all parties can be discussed. For example, the faculty member needs to know the agency's expectations of both the instructor and the nursing students. In turn, the instructor should share his or her expectations of the clinical agency. The communication of expectations before the clinical rotation commences can alleviate misunderstandings and clarify roles. There may be a registered nurse in the clinical agency that may be expected to model the role of the professional nurse. If no such nurse exists, the clinical instructor may need to fill the position of role model. Ancillary professional persons in the community setting can be identified and their roles explained at these preliminary meetings or visits. Health educators and social workers, for example, can be valuable resources to the students, assisting them in understanding the importance of collaborative, interdisciplinary relationships among health-care persons.

Initial planning may take place during these presemester planning meetings at the clinical agencies. Orientations for instructors and students can be scheduled, and details of parking and meeting places for preconferences and postconferences can be discussed. If the faculty member has ideas for teaching or learning activities for the students, these ideas may be discussed with the agency liaison. A letter of introduction to clients and/or their families may need to be approved by the agency before it is shared with clients and families. This should be accomplished as early as possible in the semester, if not before the semester, to expedite the identification of clients or families to participate in student learning experiences, if appropriate to the site.

CONTRACTS AT GMU—MY EXPERIENCE

Having taught in various clinical sites for 2 years for GMU's College of Nursing and Health Science, I was delighted to be invited to assume the position of clinical placement coordinator and community liaison. I also maintained my faculty practice in one of the largest health-care systems in Northern Virginia. These experiences greatly enhanced my familiarity with a variety of clinical agencies. However, we had only lived in Northern Virginia for approximately 5 years. Therein lay the challenge of becoming familiar with the District of Columbia and Maryland.

Luckily, the former clinical placement coordinator was able to provide me with approximately 2 weeks of orientation. I must admit a sinking feeling as I perused the 6 large black binders filled with nearly 350 contracts. The contracts were organized according to type of facility. For instance, some of the categories of facilities were hospitals, long-term care facilities, individual physician practices, and military facilities. This was an efficient system for the former placement coordinator because of her familiarity with the system and the agencies. Because I was unfamiliar with many of the organizations, I did not know how they were categorized and could not pick up the correct binder quickly.

It was clearly articulated by our dean that no student, undergraduate or graduate, would be placed in an agency without a current, valid contract in place. It was my job to find out all of the sites where our college's students were placed and determine if a valid contract was on file.

The first task was to change the filing system to alphabetical order. Next, I listed all contracts and their dates of expiration. A contract is typically valid for 3 years unless the agency requires an annual renewal. "Automatic renewal" was a term that was acceptable on the old contracts, but I was asked by our legal department to update these contracts to eliminate the automatic renewal clause.

Our legal department was most supportive in defining the legal language and explaining terms of our standard GMU contract. I also learned that the clinical agencies may initiate the agreement with their own contracts and that some change in the language of our standard contract would be acceptable. The stipulation in accepting new language was that it had to be compatible with the contracting guidelines of the Commonwealth of Virginia. The GMU legal department was available to answer my questions and was willing to answer questions directly from the community agencies.

Some of the key features of the contract are that it outlines the legal responsibilities of GMU, the college and faculty, and the agency. Another feature is that both undergraduate and graduate students are addressed. Agencies are at liberty to accept students at their own determined frequency. They are not required to accept students every semester, nor are we required to place students in specific agencies every semester.

Even though I was warned that sites do not always keep their commitments to accept students, I was dismayed when some agencies declined student placement within the first 2 weeks of my tenure in the position. Some of the agencies closed, some administrators who agreed to accept students left the organization, some organizations had downsized, and some decided that they simply could not accommodate a faculty person and students during the semester. There is no penalty for these declinations. However, it causes the greatest upset to the students. Many students choose a particular clinical site based on geographic location or other reasons. When they return after a semester break and find a change of placement assignment, it is often unsettling.

When notice is short, and students need to be placed quickly, it is ideal to use sites already under contract. However, this is not always possible. To develop a new site or to renew a contract, 3 months' time is usually required. The process is rushed if that amount of time is unrealistic. With situations such as this, it is ideal to have additional agencies under contract so that one can draw from a pool of possibilities. Some agencies do not want to contract unless student placement is imminent.

A Celebrated Contract

Perhaps my proudest achievement was securing a contract with the county health department to gain access to the county schools. The county health department employed the public health nurses that had the oversight of the school clinics. We wanted to have access to the school-age population, but found out that previously formed alliances with individual schools would no longer be sufficient. The county wanted to coordinate the work with the school children.

I called a meeting with all interested parties. Invited guests included the area school superintendent, administrators from the county health department, the dean of the College of Nursing and Health Science, the associate dean of undergraduate programs, a public health nurse and faculty member, and me. We had lunch and discussed many issues concerned with nursing students in the schools, coordination of schools used, oversight by the county health department, and, of course, the contract. What could have meant the loss of schools as clinical placement sites became the opportunity to consider more schools as placement possibilities. It was decided that the county health department would be the "gatekeeper" of nursing student placements in the county public schools.

Pitfalls to Avoid

As I already mentioned, it is very important to have more contracts on file than are needed for any single semester. Those contracts should be tagged with the types of facilities they encompass and with the level of learners that the agencies are willing to accept. For example, a physician's office may accept only nurse practitioner students, whereas an elementary school or clinic in an underserved area may welcome graduate and undergraduate learners. The pitfall would be in cutting the agency short by not considering all levels of students that may benefit from the experience.

It takes less of the administrator's time if the placement coordinators have done their homework and are familiar with the agency, its size, number of clients, and other schools and disciplines that already use the facility. The placement coordinator must understand when a placement is refused because of overcrowding. Size is also important when contracting for a site. It is unfair to send a faculty member and 10 students into a building that cannot accommodate all of them or does not have a meeting room where they can convene for preconferences and postconferences.

The most successful contract negotiations took place when I physically visited the agency. An initial phone call is a professional courtesy to briefly describe your desire for an affiliation. It is wise to ask for an appointment to discuss the school's needs and the level(s) of students that you are seeking to place. In my experience, the first reaction of agency directors was to refuse access if I had sought them out versus the agency calling me for students to come to their agency. Most administrators are very busy, at times providing care to clients and running the business. Again, it is understandable that their initial reactions would be negative. I also found that the administrators had a much more difficult time saying "no" if I was in their offices than if I was merely on the phone with them.

Another very serious pitfall is the lack of communication. Both agencies and faculty members require as much information about the other as possible. Agencies must be provided with the dates of the clinical, hours per clinical day, dates for the semester, and holidays observed by the university. Clients and staff develop relationships with the faculty members and students and need to be prepared when faculty and students will be absent.

Follow-up communication must be done after the contract is sent to the agency. The contract can look intimidating, and the administrators may hesitate to ask questions and hold up the progress of the contract. The offer of help to interpret the contract should be extended. Again, frequent communication with the potential agency will help the school administrator assess problem areas that may be of concern to the agency.

To avoid the extended delay of the progress of a contract, I found it very helpful to identify a contact person who would facilitate the signing of the contract. If the top executive received the contract, I often did not receive any feedback concerning the contract. If I was able to locate the "contract person" for the agency, the tracking of the contract was much easier. Clearly stating the expected turnaround time for the signed contract to be returned to the school is another effective strategy. Ten working days is a reasonable time frame.

Affiliate Faculty Status

When agency administrators or agency staff met the criteria for affiliate faculty status of a minimum of a master's degree and at least 8 hours of contact with the students per semester, I offered it to them. Affiliate faculty receive identification cards from GMU, free access to the university computer system, and a certificate of appreciation. Because the agency persons support our faculty and students but receive no compensation, the affiliate faculty status is one means of showing our appreciation. We value these community partnerships and would like to sustain them.

It is clear that nursing education must provide relevant student clinical experiences to prepare students to meet health-care needs in a changing society. Community-based care with a focus on health promotion and disease prevention in a holistic approach is to be emphasized. Collaboration with other health team members in non-traditional clinical settings enhances the effective preparation of future nurse professionals (Giltinan 1998).

As competition for community-based sites increases because health-care educators recognize the need for better preparation of students in community sites, it behooves nurse educators and administrators to pay attention to detail in working to secure community-based sites and contracts. Locating, negotiating, maintaining, and evaluating community-based experiences will be an ongoing process. Administrators will need to negotiate clinical contracts as placements are needed. Flexibility is imperative given the ever-changing situations in the community (De La Garza & Martinez-Rogers 1998). Perhaps it is even more important to continually communicate both needs and expectations of the nursing program and the agencies throughout the semesters and years of the affiliation to maintain positive and truly mutually beneficial relationships.

References

Armentrout, G (1998). Community based nursing. Foundation for practice. Stamford, CT: Appleton & Lange.

De La Garza, S, & Martinez-Rogers, N (1998). Community clinical sites for psychiatric nursing students. J Nurs Educ 37(3):142-143.

Gaither, L, et al. (1998). Service-Learning Handbook, Faculty Edition. Center for Service and Leadership, Fairfax, VA: George Mason University.

Giltinan, JM (1998). A veterans affairs facility provides independent home-health clinical experiences with a case manager focus. J Nurs Educ 37(3):136-138.

Gray, LK, et al. (1998). A community health practicum model for baccalaureate nursing students. Home Care Provid 3(2):105-110.

Greenberg, JS (1999). Service learning in health education. College of Health & Human Performance, Baltimore, MD: University of Maryland, Spring.

Noble, MA, et al. (1996). Shifting the educational paradigm for the nurse of tomorrow: A community-focused curriculum. N HC Perspect Community 17, 66-71.

Webster's New Basic Dictionary (1997). Promotional Sales Books, LLC.

Yoder, MH, et al. (1997). Agency-university collaboration: Home care early in the student curriculum. Home Healthcare Nurse 15(7): 493-499.

Zotti, ME, et al. (1996). Community-based nursing versus community health nursing: What does it all mean? Nurs Outlook 44:211-217.

CHAPTER 2

Selection of Faculty for a Community-based Curriculum

Margaret A. Miklancie

Learning Objectives

1) Discuss how potential faculty are interviewed and what qualities are desirable.

2) Examine important values needed by nurse educators in a community-based curriculum.

3) Describe important characteristics of community-based educators.

4) Analyze components of successful experiences though "lessons learned."

Table 2-1

GMU's College of Nursing and Health Sciences Faculty Positions

George Mason University College of Nursing and Health Science is seeking part-time teaching and clinical faculty for Fall and Spring semesters.
MSN required. Prior teaching experience preferred.
Must be enthusiastic, caring, and creative.
Must have love of teaching and learning.
Strong communication skills required.
Must have working knowledge of community health.
Health promotion and disease prevention concepts a must.
Professional role modeling required.

Send letter of application and curriculum vita to:
Margaret A. Miklancie, RN, PhD
Coordinator, Undergraduate Nursing Program
George Mason University
College of Nursing & Health Science
MSN 3 C 4
4400 University Drive
Fairfax, Virginia 22030-4444
703-993-1927 AA/EEO

Sounds like a tall order to fill? Listen to the story of Anna who applied to George Mason University (GMU) to teach in our community-based program. The available position was supervising nursing students in an elementary school, identified as a "special needs" school serving children and families from vulnerable and underserved areas in Fairfax County.

Anna's nursing practice background was in pediatrics, and most currently pediatric emergency room experience. Anna also worked with nursing students in the past in community-based sites. Anna seemed to have a command of teaching learning principles when responding to questions dealing with challenging students and how to best assist them in meeting their educational learning objectives. Anna said all the right answers, seemed confident in her nursing practice and future teaching opportunity at GMU. Nine weeks into the semester, Anna resigned. What happened?

The second applicant was Katrina. The available position was supervising nursing students in an HIV services department of a local community hospital in the northern

Virginia area serving vulnerable and underserved persons in Fairfax County.

> Katrina's nursing practice background was as an Adult Nurse Practitioner and most currently serving the needs of HIV clients where she was employed. Katrina never taught in a formal way in a university setting. Katrina had served as a preceptor for graduate students and implemented several in-service education programs for groups of HIV positive clients.
>
> Katrina seemed to have a command of teaching-learning principles when responding to questions dealing with challenging students and how to best assist them in meeting their educational learning objectives. Katrina responded with many of the right answers, seemed confident in her nursing practice and future teaching opportunity at GMU.
>
> Katrina received glowing student evaluations at the end of the 16 weeks. She is now enjoying her second semester teaching at GMU. Why? What made the difference between these two seemingly competent individuals?

This chapter will explore the fundamentals of choosing faculty for a community-based site. I will outline what comprises selection criteria for potential faculty, explore characteristics and values of individual faculty members, and share some lessons learned from working with part-time faculty.

Let's begin with two assumptions that I believe to be true of all nurse educators:

- Faculty in nursing programs share common professional values in nursing education whether they are in an associate degree or a baccalaureate degree program. For example, "The Essentials of Baccalaureate Education for Professional Nursing Practice" (American Association of Colleges of Nursing—AACN 1998) defines values as "beliefs or ideals to which an individual is committed and which are reflected in patterns of behavior. Professional values are the foundation for practice; they guide interactions with patients, colleagues, other professionals, and the public" (p 8). Among the values that we share in teaching are caring, altruism, autonomy, human dignity, integrity, and social justice.
- Nursing faculty are cognizant of the collaborative and interdisciplinary nature of the health-care arenas, be they acute care or community-based in nature.

SELECTION CRITERIA FOR POTENTIAL FACULTY

The process of recruiting and interviewing faculty is fairly common at all institutions. GMU is an Equal Opportunity Employer, and each qualified person who applies for a position does have an opportunity to be interviewed (George Mason University, 1996).

In recruiting faculty for the community-based sites, knowledge of community health nursing and community resources are strongly preferred. However, this is not to say that one without community nursing experience will not be successful. Faculty development was an important topic when the College of Nursing and Health Science moved to a community-based curriculum (CBC) in 1994. Our full-time faculty members, with an exclusive orientation to acute-care settings, became retooled to function in a community-based curriculum. The process was a challenging but successful one. Specific aspects of faculty development will be integrated and addressed in "lessons learned" sections.

The Interview

Usually the interview session lasts from 1 hour to 1 hour and 15 minutes. This is usually sufficient time to learn about the person's nursing background, areas of expertise, teaching backgrounds, experiences with culturally diverse groups, and nursing philosophy. An opportunity to share how GMU's curriculum is laid out is important, be-

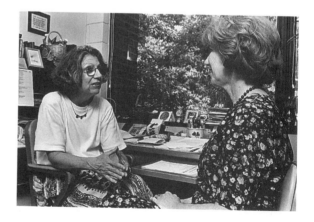

cause ours is not a conventionally structured curriculum. The profile of our students is shared.

If the applicant has teaching experience, I ask him or her to tell me about a particularly challenging student he or she dealt with and the final outcome. If the applicant does not have experience, I pose several scenarios that may be encountered while working with students, and ask how he or she would handle each one. There usually are no right and wrong ways to answer; rather, I hear different approaches that may tell me how creative and inventive the candidate will be as a faculty member.

I like to have applicants share a favorite story from their nursing practice that depicts caring, explain how this story might have changed them as a person and as a nurse, and relate the implications for their nursing practice. This gives insight into how they will be able to enter into creating a caring environment for nursing students.

We also talk about values in nursing education and the impact of role modeling for nursing students. Many can remember stories of strong role models in their past educational experiences and the power those hold for them, even to this day.

Finally, we talk about the site itself, the importance of knowing the community-based site, the resources available in the community, the teaching-learning principles, how they might stimulate critical thinking in the students, the requirements of the course, and how they can assist students in meeting and exceeding the objectives of the course.

The applicant leaves knowing what paperwork is required to qualify for a position. In fairness to each person, I sit down immediately after the interview and summarize salient points, capitalizing on the strengths of the person, how he or she might handle certain situations, and my overall impressions. Many times in the process of the interview, I learn about other strengths and talents where the person's expertise may be used in the curriculum. Recommendations are made on behalf of the candidates to the associate dean for the undergraduate programs, who collaborates with me in the decision-making process to choose the *best* candidates for the available positions to be filled.

The next section will explore professional values. Nurse educators who choose nursing education as a career

---

Table 2-2

Sample Interview Questions

Faculty with prior teaching experience

1. From your previous teaching experiences, can you site an example for me of a particularly challenging student situation you encountered? Tell me what the essence of the scenario was, how you handled the particular situation, and what the final outcome of the scenario was, be it positive or otherwise.

Faculty without teaching experience

I will pose several scenarios to you. I would like you to tell me how you would handle each one.

1. A student arrives late for preconference for the second day in a row. The first day this happened, you overlooked the tardiness.

2. All of your students except one are actively engaged with their clients. You notice that the student apparently is stalling by reading a pamphlet that could possibly wait until the clients leave. Tell me how you would approach this particular student.

Table 2-2 (continued)

3. One student is having difficulty applying the nursing process to his or her current client, despite several group postconference times dedicated to this topic. How would you creatively help this student grasp the concept in a meaningful way?

have a special set of values and characteristics that they hold in their belief system that adds to excellence in nursing education.

Professional Values of Community-based Educators

I believe that values are important considerations in selection of faculty. Faculty values are likely to affect which values they try to develop in students. I will address some of these attributes based on the current AACN's Essentials document. (AACN 1998).

Professional Values

Nursing education should facilitate the development of professional values and value-based behaviors (AACN 1998). *The Random House Dictionary* (1989) defines *values* as "ideals or principles, as of a given society, to regard highly" (p 961).

The nursing community holds certain ideals upon which future nurses build their practice philosophy. Attributes such as ethical thinking, promise keeping, truth telling, following through, caring, commitment, and excellent communication skills are among the many values that professionals hold. These values can be assimilated if they are part of the students' education as they build their philosophy of nursing practice.

Values in Our History

Providing safe humanistic care to each person dates back to Florence Nightingale. Florence became so involved in the hospital administration and in preparing nurses to care for the wounded in battle, she was unable to make her rounds until the early hours of the morning. She visited patients carrying her lamp. She talked to them and saw them as whole persons. Her presence was a way to demonstrate each one's value. Working nurses, on a daily basis, create this same atmosphere. Experts can give humanistic care without thinking. Novice nurses must contemplate each step of the process.

Current Thinking on Values

The AACN (1998) refers to the attribute of *altruism* as the concern for the welfare of each client, colleague, and other health-care provider. In our society today, altruism embraces cultural competence. *Cultural competence* allows nurses to meet the client where they are perhaps grounded in different values, and to meet the health-care needs of the individual and family as a unit. Altruism includes acting as the client's advocate at all times, especially when his or her voice cannot be heard. Finally, experienced nurses have a responsibility to mentor new nurses because they too were mentored and coached along the way.

Another value is respect for the dignity of each human person. Many students enter nursing with a sense of their own dignity already inherent in their personal value system. Others develop this value in the nursing program.

Some student nurses initially have a distaste for the most vulnerable people—those poor in health, poor in material possessions, poor in spirit, and poor in coping skills for daily living. With strong faculty role models, students can learn compassion and respect for human dignity.

Protecting clients' confidentiality is an aspect of respect for human dignity.

Helping students to recognize another's value as a human being is an important role for the faculty. Each person deserves respect and dignity just because he or she is a human being. Encouraging nonjudgmental behavior is important for faculty to teach and role model. This kind of teaching occurs when nursing faculty take the time to discuss students' learning experiences even in the midst of confusion and uncertainty. Faculty must encourage every student to form and broaden his or her own value system.

Faculty play an important role in fostering discussions that heighten students' sensitivity to others. Promoting respect for each individual and the integrity of that person is paramount to promoting respect and integrity in the nursing profession.

Values of Individual Faculty Members

In reflecting upon the values of a faculty member, I will frame five specific values using Roach's (1992) five "Cs". I will look at her definitions and expand on each of them as they relate to essential faculty values. The five Cs are Commitment, Competency, Confidence, Compassion, and Conscience.

Chapter 2 | Selection of Faculty for a Community-based Curriculum

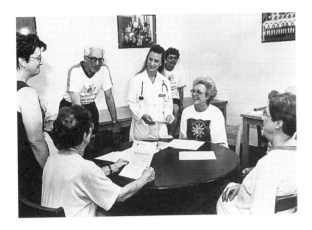

Commitment

Roach (1992) defines commitment as a "complex affective response characterized by a convergence between one's desires and one's obligations, and by a deliberate choice to act in accordance with them" (p 65). For example, at 3 a.m., a mother does not have to think about whether she should respond to the needs of her sick child. The response of the mother is an unquestionable convergence between what she wants to do (sleep) and what she needs to do (tend to her sick child).

In assessing commitment in nursing faculty, Roach's definition applies. The positive attitude of a faculty member to go above and beyond to facilitate learning experiences for nursing students permeates clinical education.

Members of other disciplines such as social work, psychology, or medicine are also faced with coaching students in formulating values. An interdisciplinary strategy such as discussion groups with other disciplines for first-year students could help everyone. Accepting and appreciating what each discipline offers is a learned process.

Many scenarios in community-based settings offer no nursing role models for our students. In such cases, the nurse faculty member is the nursing role model but may select the social worker or a physical therapist to be an effective model for the student. This provides a rich experience, both for the student and the other health-care provider. Stimulating students to identify the "role of nursing" is one of the challenges in non-nursing community-based settings for the nurse educator. The following demonstrates this example and one instructor's value of commitment.

 Delores, a faculty member, persuaded the director of a senior center (a non-nurse) to allow nursing students to visit and talk to the clients participating at the center. The concept of nursing was tied to a "feeling of sickness" in the director's mind, which made the students appear out of place. Clients coming to the center were healthy and the center's staff didn't want the clients to feel any differently about themselves.

Initially, the students felt ignored and unwanted, but gradually, one by one, the students began to form relationships with individual clients just by smiling and sitting close by. Soon, the clients were sharing important information about their lives, their families, their health, and their need for more information on their medications, diet, exercise, and blood pressure readings.

The students organized a "health fair" based on the needs expressed by the clients to answer their questions. The health fair served as a social occasion and a means of health promotion.

At the end of the semester, the clients had a farewell party for the students. The director gradually recognized the contributions of the students and asked that her senior center be included among settings for future nursing students.

This particular faculty member was able to help students to identify nursing roles within the setting. By her persistence, role modeling, and commitment to the students in this situation, it turned out to be a win-win situation. Delores was committed to go beyond the barriers initially in place and find the role of nursing in this community-based site among a healthy population.

Competency

Roach (1992) defines competency as the "state of having knowledge, judgment, skills, energy, experience, and motivation to respond adequately to the demands of one's professional responsibilities" (p 61). Roach says that historically some believe the major requirements of being a professional are kindness and physical strength. However, current thinking requires much more of health-care professionals. Nurses must hold a high degree of cognitive, affective, technical, and administrative leadership skills to be competent practitioners.

Nurse educators must be able to incorporate critical thinking, principles of pathology and pathophysiology, adult health, life span development, and recognition of legal, and political issues, insurance laws, and nurse practice acts. Masters-prepared educators usually hold broader views as a result of graduate education. Excellence in nursing education occurs when faculty can discuss and model these qualities for students. One example of this is illustrated in the following story.

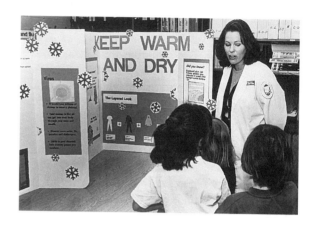

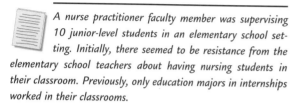

A nurse practitioner faculty member was supervising 10 junior-level students in an elementary school setting. Initially, there seemed to be resistance from the elementary school teachers about having nursing students in their classroom. Previously, only education majors in internships worked in their classrooms.

The role of the student nurse was unclear in the classroom settings. The role of the student nurse was not to tutor a child in reading or math, unless the tutoring led to establishing a therapeutic relationship. This relationship became a vehicle for identifying a health-care need to help the child. The nursing faculty member needed to work intently with the elementary school faculty to change this mindset. The nursing faculty's relationship with the classroom teachers and with the nursing students facilitated the creation of a health-oriented role in the classroom.

The faculty member also supervised the students who spent a week with the school health aide in the school's infirmary. In Virginia, school nurses have clusters of schools that are within their realm of responsibility. Each school operates within specific guidelines. The role of the school aide is delineated: when to call parents or seek medical intervention is spelled out.

A student nurse was assigned to the infirmary, and a sick child came in to be seen. The student nurse assessed the child's condition and verified her assessment with the faculty member. She made recommendations to the school health aide for an action plan. The school health aide seemed relieved that professional nursing was on hand, and that she did not have to make all the decisions. The students began to gain credibility. Teachers began stopping the nursing faculty in the hallway for consultation about students in the classroom. Students grew into the role of nurses, and teachers realized the value in having the nursing students in their classroom. Gradually, the teachers relinquished their health lessons to the nursing students. Nursing students began teaching health lessons on a daily basis.

Administratively, the faculty member demonstrated her competence and expertise in nursing, orchestrating skills to communicate with the principal and classroom teachers. The ability to attend the elementary school faculty meetings and be on the agenda was important in assisting the elementary school faculty to see the role of the nursing student. The faculty member worked with each teacher. She paved the way for the nursing students. Additionally, her competency as a nursing professional, grounded in a solid knowledge base, made her a credible member of the elementary school, collaboratively working with other disciplines.

Confidence

Promoting trusting relationships is the way Roach (1992) describes confidence. Specifically, Roach says "caring confidence fosters trust without dependency; communicates truth without violence; and creates a relationship of respect without paternalism or without engendering a response born out of fear or powerlessness. Confidence, then, is a critical attribute of professional caring" (p 63).

Faculty confidence is an important resource for students. Elements of risk-taking are necessary to be creative and to approach situations in different ways. Helping students meet the objectives of the course and have fun in the process produces wonderful outcomes when the faculty member is confident in himself or herself and in the students. One faculty member illustrates an example of confidence in the following scenario:

While visiting a faculty member and her group of students in an outpatient psychiatric center, I was struck with delight because the students were so engaged with the clients and activities happening in the center. On that particular day, the students were hosting a St. Patrick's Day party for the clients. There was singing and dancing and refreshments to mark the festive event! Sometimes, psychiatric settings can be scary for novice students, especially for the younger student. When reflecting this to the faculty member and exploring how she prepares students to function in this setting, she shared some teaching strategies:

"One of the most important aspects is that we talk a lot. In preconference and postconference and throughout the day, I'm always asking the students, what do you think? Tell me more— and I am consistently debriefing the process of what's happening with the students."

After building a trusting relationship with their clients, students are expected to take a history and perform a physical assessment. The assessment allows the student to identify areas for health promotion and teaching opportunities with the client. Some students are uncomfortable with this aspect.

After a period of grooming I know the students are ready to do their physical assessment, but the students don't know they are ready. I tell them, 'You'll do fine. Sit and listen. Tell them your expectations. Follow the client's lead.' I love the students with a servant's heart because they live up to all they can become. Students, in turn, find their clients fulfill their expectations.

When faculty are confident, students are generally confident. The faculty member instills this characteristic as she or he role models for the students. When the faculty members are confident in their roles and skills as nurses and educators, they can be a marvelous influence on the students' progress and development.

In interviewing faculty who apply to work in our program, I explore this area with them by asking them some questions.

Box 2-1 Learning Exercise for Faculty Use

Faculty Confidence

How do you use your own skills and abilities to promote student confidence?

How do you deal with a student who is extremely shy?

What do you do to facilitate teamwork among the students?

In all situations, truth and trusting relationships are the building blocks on which to stimulate students to be risk takers and tap into the resources within themselves and to be resources for each other.

Compassion

Compassion is defined as a "way of living out an awareness of one's relationship to all living creatures: engendering a response of participation in the experience of another; a sensitivity to the pain and brokenness of the other; a quality of presence which allows one to share with and make room for the other" (Roach 1992, p 58). There may be some authors who feel that compassion can be taught, like taking a temperature or blood pressure. Other authors (Fox 1990, Fox & Sheldrake1996, Nouwen, et al. 1982) feel it is a gift.

Certain individuals come into the profession because they are compassionate. This quality seems to be inherent in nursing students. Some may have a greater capacity to become more compassionate. Can this capacity be increased through nursing education? I believe that it can. Every day in the courses, clinicals, and classrooms in which we interact with students and colleagues, there are many opportunities to teach compassion.

In my own teaching experience, I can recall instances of compassion I did not know possible.

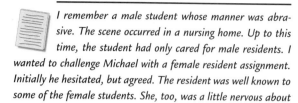

> I remember a male student whose manner was abrasive. The scene occurred in a nursing home. Up to this time, the student had only cared for male residents. I wanted to challenge Michael with a female resident assignment. Initially he hesitated, but agreed. The resident was well known to some of the female students. She, too, was a little nervous about a male student caring for her daily needs.
>
> With reassurance that other students and myself would be available to assist, the resident agreed.
>
> A surprise outcome occurred. Initially, the resident and student nurse seemed to get along together cordially. Because I was involved with the needs of the other students, it was a while before I was able to get back to that room. To my surprise, the resident had been given a shower and shampoo. She was wearing a good dress and jewelry, and Michael was applying her makeup when I entered the room. His next step was to file and paint her fingernails.
>
> Michael's compassionate side, once he was open to it, became visible elsewhere, too—in the nursery, holding and feeding newborn babies, working with a woman dying from lung cancer, and interacting with his peers and staff members. I believe Michael may not have been given planned opportunities by other faculty to be compassionate. He was labeled unfairly.

When faculty are compassionate, caring occurs naturally. When faculty are compassionate with students, trust is strengthened in the relationship. When faculty demonstrate compassion, students learn from their compassion.

Conscience

Conscience is defined as "a state of moral awareness: a compass directing one's behavior according to the moral fitness of things" (Roach 1992, p 63). "Conscience is neither innate, nor is it simply a thing added on at some point in one's experience. Conscience grows out of a process of valuing self and others. Conscience is the call of care and manifests itself as care" (p 64).

In valuing the nursing student, the faculty member does so in a variety of ways. The first way is to actively listen to the student, attempting to understand the student so he or she really feels heard. Students often have many feelings going on at any given time. To be able to assist students to clarify, amplify, and verify their feelings takes a faculty member who is available and can listen through the words or silence to the thoughts and feelings expressed.

One illustration to highlight this is a story about a visiting professor who was asked to go into a math class for the hour period.

> One young man sat at the far back corner of the classroom, cap over his eyes and with no notebook or writing instrument handy. His behavior suggested boredom and displeasure. The professor tried to draw out the young man, but to no avail. The professor dismissed the class feeling that he had failed because of his inability to connect with this student or motivate him to participate in the class session.
>
> Later that afternoon, the visiting professor was scheduled to return to his home across the nation. A driver showed up to take him to the airport. To his surprise, the driver was none other than the disinterested student who sat in his class earlier in the day. As the professor began to engage the young man in conversation, he learned more than he could have imagined.
>
> The young man shared how his father was an alcoholic and his mother, deceased. He needed to work to provide basic necessities for the family plus to finish school. The young man started to weep. The professor took the time to listen to his story and suddenly understood why the youth had no energy for his course work. The young man was physically exhausted.
>
> The young man asked to speak with this professor in the future. Though not the professor's normal mode of operation, he gave his phone number to the young man and for the longest time, they kept in touch.
>
> The moral compass of this professor led him to act in a healing manner to assist this young man. The professor valued the young man and demonstrated this in taking an interest in his life. He acted in an ethical way. Perhaps he was the only male role model this student had ever known (Palmer 1998).

In nursing, faculty use their conscience on a daily basis. One nursing faculty member does this by creating a safe environment where each student's opinion is voiced and valued. Another faculty member gives thoughtful, lengthy written feedback in student journals. Another has worked with a student recently diagnosed with cancer. Yet another creative faculty member writes "prescriptions of care" to assist the students in technology lab.

In summary, I have discussed professional values defined by AACN as essentials in nursing education. Roach's classification of Commitment, Competency, Confidence, Compassion, and Conscience serve as a values framework for selection of excellent faculty members. The next section will address salient characteristics required for successful educators working in a community-based settings with nursing students.

Characteristics of Excellence in Community-based Educators

"Excellent teachers have one thing in common—a passion to keep improving their abilities. One does not just arrive at being an expert teacher. The drive towards excellence is an ongoing process that continues throughout the teacher's entire professional life" (Bastable 1997, p 280). The following seven characteristics are proposed as a framework for excellence in selecting faculty for community-based settings. I will end this section with one faculty member's story which combines many of these qualities.

Command of the Content and Knowledge of the Community Setting

Faculty need to have an operational command of the setting to which they take students. Faculty may do this in a variety of ways, one of which is by being employed in the setting on a part-time basis so that they gain familiarity with the organization on a personal level. A second way is to spend 2 or 3 days in the setting, becoming oriented to policies and procedures, and becoming familiar with the staff.

In selecting faculty for community-based settings, command of content areas such as gerontology or chronic care may be invaluable even though they may not be formally prepared in community health. It is essential, however, that they understand community resources and how to integrate specialized content areas into the community setting.

In the beginning, when our faculty were transitioning to the community-based curriculum, it was important for them to be familiar with the setting and how best to function. The community health faculty served as the guides and mentors in orienting faculty from primarily acute-care settings to become more familiar and comfortable in assuming the new community health role.

Promoting wellness and preventing disease took on a greater importance to all the faculty. Solid knowledge in adult health nursing is paramount. Growth and development across the life span and maternal and pediatric information are critical areas in the community. In the first year, faculty and students learned together.

Excellent Communication Skills

Strong communication is an essential element of faculty function both in and out of community-based sites, particularly interdisciplinary communication. Initially, persons from the administrative faculty are the first contact people. Meetings are held to explore options for the students. Once the path is cleared, faculty are given names of contacts in the agencies, and they begin to work directly with those contacts. Faculty start weeks ahead to explore the community. The role of the student nurse is explained and highlighted. The mission and philosophy of the college is shared.

Faculty meet with the key players. The course description and objectives are shared with all involved. A variety of ways in which students can meet the objectives are brainstormed with staff. Successful achievement in the setting requires that *all* involved in the student's educational experience have the information.

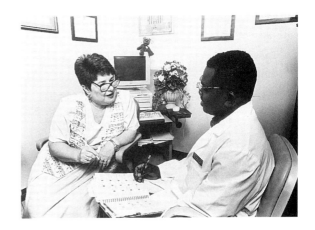

In the first year of our community-based program, we learned many lessons about communication which helped us set standards and policies in the years since. One faculty member was supervising students who were spread throughout three different sites. The faculty member was ill one week. She kept her beeper turned on at home and communicated with the students by phone when questions or problems were presented. There were no preconferences or postconferences that week. This faculty member did not understand the importance of physical visibility and being available to the students. We quickly established "Guidelines for Clinical Supervison in Community-based Sites" (see Chap. 1, Table 1–4).

Enthusiasm about Teaching and Nursing

Faculty who are invested in teaching and have a passion for nursing have a way to excite students. This enthusiasm comes across with high energy in committing to the educational experiences with the students. No matter how knowledgeable the educator is about the site and the content of the course, if he or she is unable to communicate this with enthusiasm, it will fall on deaf ears. Enthusiasm is contagious. Students marvel at themselves and how differently they feel about the course or the clinical experience.

Risk Taking

Risk-taking faculty often have a strong intuition and rely on that as a compass to guide them in situations with the students. Faculty who can present examples of different scenarios to students and allow students to brainstorm with each other help in three ways:

1. They allow the students to tap into their own internal resources to solve problems.
2. They give students permission to extend themselves and make mistakes. We need to allow this process to play itself out, unless, of course, safety is an issue. Faculty need to be present to students, and help them pick up the pieces if they are not successful.
3. They allow students and faculty members to enter into true partnerships in the educational endeavor. We learn to take risks by taking them and critically evaluating the results.

Sense of Humor

Effective teachers use humor to get the attention of the students. Humor that is appropriate has the ability to unite the group and bring a humanness to the faculty member. Current literature indicates that the therapeutic effects of using humor have a direct link to and benefit the whole body by releasing endorphins. Humor, however, is not used at another's expense. The ability to laugh at oneself or the situation allows one to make mistakes without embarrassment and gives students the freedom to experiment with other learning methods.

Role Modeling

Effective faculty are role models for students on several different levels. First, actions *do* speak louder than words, and students may mimic the behaviors that they wish to emulate. Second, faculty who have a thirst to keep abreast of the latest research, theory, and clinical and community issues can facilitate meaningful discussions with students. Faculty are likely to instill this zest for lifelong learning in their students as future professionals. Current information and research findings integrated into discussions with students add to the faculty member's credibility. The third level concerns the students' internal locus of control, tapping into their own resources to build character and endurance, including mental, emotional, psychological, and spiritual strengths. Students can be taught how to mobilize these qualities by faculty whom they admire. Modeling for the students is one of the most important ways we can teach.

Creativity

Creativity is looking and coloring outside traditional boundaries. The creative teacher is one who sees unlimited possibilities in different situations and helps the student to see them too. Nurses have always been good at finding ways to meet the needs of the clients in unconventional ways. Creativity in students is an area that can be developed and enhanced with creative faculty.

One example that illustrates creativity and many other characteristics we've discussed follows.

> Mary's clinical group was made up of a diverse student population. Many students were quiet, shy, or unfamiliar with taking the lead. The parish setting in which the students worked provided opportunities for nursing students to work with clients across the life span.
>
> In the elementary school of this parish, the faculty member facilitated an "International Health Fair" with her 10 diverse clinical students. Students wore the traditional garb of their countries. Each chose a health promotion facet of interest to elementary school children, which included bike safety, poison alerts, and exercise. Tables were set up with native foods and nutritional tidbits of information to assist the elementary school children with healthy choices. One highlight of the whole experience was the elementary students seeing the nursing student dressed in his or her native garb.
>
> The elementary school children had a "health passport." As children went to each table or booth, their passports were stamped. After visiting all the booths, rewards were given to each child. The incentives to have all the passports stamped, as well as the experience of learning about healthy bodies, made the health promotion activity fun for the children. The nursing students learned the joy of teaching-learning in creative ways. Through the creativity of this faculty member, planting the seeds of ingenuity and flexibility, the nursing students were able to make a positive contribution to the health of the elementary school children.

This project took all semester to plan, orchestrate, implement, and evaluate. The students researched information that was age appropriate. They needed to locate community resources and obtain materials that could be integrated into their project or handed out at the health fair. The nursing students communicated with the teachers and elementary students. They also prepared a letter to be sent home to parents. The students were excited, and this spilled over to the children with whom they were working. Children bring a joy and sense of humor to every situation. I have found that nursing students have this ability as well.

The clinical faculty member used the strengths of the group to the best possible advantage. Influencing cultural competency while promoting health and wellness in elementary school students is a challenge. The secret ingredient was the relevancy for both student groups, which contributed to making the experience an enjoyable one.

Educators need to be aware of changing student needs in nursing education today. Students come with rich resources. Many have second degrees. Many have past or current real-world working experience. Some manage families, are single parents, and orchestrate households. All hold great value for nursing. These facts are important to remember when interacting with students and assisting them to grow to their full potential.

In summary, I have explored additional characteristics of excellent faculty members, namely those who have command of nursing content and of the community site; have strong communications skills, great enthusiasm, a sense of humor, and risk-taking abilities; role model for students; and are creative and flexible in their current responsibilities. Lessons learned are based on our experience.

LESSONS LEARNED

We now turn to Anna and Katrina. Do you have any speculations about why Anna resigned and Katrina is still employed? Let's explore aspects of both situations.

Both faculty members met the qualifications to be hired in the College of Nursing and Health Science.

Both faculty members received an orientation to the college and the course. Both seemed to have a good understanding of the faculty expectations and role.

Although both faculty members were expert in their specialty area, Anna had mastered working with ill children but did not seem to know how to guide nursing students in the promotion of health and wellness with children. Katrina's approach to the HIV population was focused on maintenance and promotion of wellness to the maximum level. She was able to share this perspective with the students she was working with in the setting.

Anna initially came across as quiet and reserved and presented herself in the most professional way. Despite the fact that Anna had a cell phone, beeper, and fax at home to receive student assignments, she was not a good communicator. Anna seemed awkward in communicating important information to the students, staff, and key persons in the college. Katrina, on the other hand, had only the beeper as her main tool (which is provided through the college to all clinical faculty). She was a visual communicator and used the written word to strengthen and amplify materials that were important. Another difference was Anna's lack of enthusiasm. Initially, I interpreted the situation as Anna being overwhelmed with all the information of a new job. What I learned later was that Anna was enrolled in three graduate classes, worked part-time at the hospital, and worked with our nursing students. The impact of her low energy level and lack of enthusiasm was difficult to overcome by the second faculty member who took over the site when Anna resigned. I believe Anna modeled this negative attitude to the students, and they too became skeptics.

I learned two unfortunate lessons from this experience—first, "the see for myself" approach. When I or the course coordinator kept in daily telephone contact with Anna on clinical days, she always reassured us, "we're doing fine" and "there are no questions right now." It was not until I visited the faculty member around week 6 that I realized the complexity of the situation. I now realize that new faculty need the support of administration much earlier in the rotation.

Second, a "fine line" exists in mentoring, especially when you are working with a faculty member with prior teaching experience. Knowing when the faculty member needs help and when to back off takes some intuition.

Since my experience with Anna, I try to use intuition to guide me in the decision-making process when selecting and orienting new faculty. One of the roles I have in the college is to visit the newly hired faculty member and group of students at the clinical agency. Primarily, I am there to assist and mentor the faculty in the day-to-day activities with the students. In the process of going through the day with the faculty, many questions are answered, and usually there is time for clarification. It is also a special time to see the students in action and get to know them. There have been times when I attended the first-day orientation at an agency with the faculty and students. Being with the new faculty is a good way to offer support and answer questions that new faculty and students may have. It also gives me the opportunity to hear the same information that the students are hearing. I then return in several weeks to again spend the day or part of the day with faculty and students. This is time well spent in the long run. Stabilizing the foundation, pointing out to faculty what they are doing well, and addressing other ways to accomplish activities assist the new faculty member in his or her development as an excellent educator.

I always try to make time to meet with the key persons at the agency to get their perspective of the students' progress and faculty in general. Expectations can be clarified during this conversation. It provides an opportunity to thank the agency staff for allowing our students to come and meet their learning objectives. We value our community partners, and the partnership can be strengthened during this interaction.

Selecting faculty to work and guide nursing students in community-based sites presents opportunities and challenges. The opportunity to develop the potential of new faculty in nursing education is exciting, knowing they will play important roles in shaping the profession in the future. Careful selection of faculty and their effective development is necessary for effective development of students.

References

American Association of Colleges of Nursing (1998). The essentials of baccalaureate education for professional nursing practice. Washington, DC: AACN.

Bastable, SB (1997). Nurse as educator: Principles of teaching and learning. Sudbury, MA: Jones & Bartlett.

Fox, M (1990). A spirituality named compassion. San Francisco: Harper Collins.

Fox, M, and Sheldrake, R (1996). Natural grace. New York: Doubleday.

George Mason University (1996). Wage Employees Orientation (Workshop). Fairfax, VA: George Mason University, August 25.

Nouwen, HJM, et al. (1982). Compassion: A reflection on the Christian life. New York: Doubleday.

Palmer, PJ (1998). The courage to teach: Exploring the inner landscape of a teacher's life. San Francisco: Jossey-Bass.

Random House Webster's College Dictionary, 2nd ed. (2000). New York: Random House.

Roach, S (1992). The human act of caring: A blueprint for the health professions. Ottawa, Canada: Canadian Hospital Association Press.

CHAPTER 3

Teaching through Stories: An Approach to Student-centered Learning

Jeanne M. Sorrell

Learning Objectives

1) Describe the value of using stories for student-centered learning.
2) Differentiate the use of case studies from narratives as a teaching strategy in nursing.
3) Discuss outcomes of composition research that relate to storytelling as a teaching strategy.
4) Discuss the use of storytelling as a teaching strategy in the nursing classroom and community-based clinical experiences.
5) Discuss strategies for helping students to compose effective stories.
6) Identify approaches for evaluating students' stories.

I remember vividly the first time I decided to use stories as a major part of my course. At the first class period of the semester, I reviewed the syllabus with the students and told them that the course assignments included the writing of two stories: one about their own experience and one from a client's point of view. I saw some students in the back rolling their eyes, especially when I told them that they would need to interview one of their clients about the "lived experience" of living with an illness. I began to have second thoughts about whether I really wanted to go through with this!—Author

The opening story illustrates the anxiety that often comes with implementing a major change in a teaching approach. I taught for many years and was happy with students' responses to my teaching. Students seemed to enjoy my classes and rated them highly. As the content that I was expected to "cover" in the classes became more and more complex, however, it became increasingly difficult to find ways to help the students understand this content. In my intent to *cover* the required content, I realized that I sometimes covered over, or obscured, the most important understandings I wanted the students to gain.

Stories emerged as an approach to *uncover* these understandings for students in my classes. I believe that the use of stories offers a unique teaching approach that helps to uncover understandings that are critical for students to grasp as they prepare for roles in community-based nursing practice.

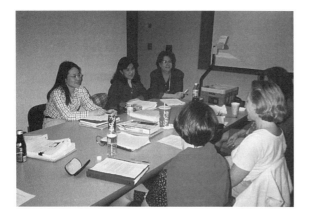

TEACHING WITH STORIES

As nursing education enters the 21st century, many nurse educators are looking to new pedagogies to prepare students for new, increasingly complex roles in community-based nursing practice. Pedagogies are needed that foster critical thinking and caring behaviors through student-centered learning approaches (Sorrell 2001). Stories offer important possibilities for meeting these desired learning outcomes. Geanellos (1996) states that nurses' stories help them to reconstruct the essence of important experiences. Learning to listen and to hear the core truth of a story is a critical skill for nurses to acquire. When stories of teacher and student are shared together, it creates a unique pedagogical experience.

Van Manen (1991) conceptualizes "curriculum" as comprising the structures and phases of study at an educational institution. In contrast, he views "pedagogy" as a concept embodied by human, interpersonal, and caring processes of education. Van Manen describes pedagogy as a process that "draws us caringly" toward those whom we teach (p 31). The "pedagogical moment" emerges as an important concept in this approach to teaching (p 40). Van Manen defines the pedagogical moment as the point of active encounter between teacher and student, an opportunity for the teacher to initiate a transformational learning interaction experienced by the student as caring (p 130).

The following story illustrates how storytelling as a teaching strategy can create unexpected and transformational learning experiences:

 I was exploring with my students the different characteristics of novice and expert nurses and wanted them to have the experience of talking with an expert nurse. Diane agreed to meet with us for our postconference. As an oncology clinical nurse specialist, she was the epitome of the expert clinician. She had the reputation of being the "clin-spec of clin-specs" among her peers, with a no-nonsense approach to the management of complex cases. I looked forward to hearing her sophisticated analysis of her advanced practice role.

I told the students that they should facilitate the session; I would stay in the background. After some preliminary discussion about how Diane approached the complex problems in her expert role, one of the students asked her to tell a story about an experience from her practice that stood out in her mind. Diane's surprise was evident, and she hesitated. I, too, became somewhat anxious at this unexpected turn in our conference and wondered whether I should step in. But then I heard Diane begin her story.

We listened intently as Diane told us of a 4-year-old boy, Terry, who was with his mother at home when she died after a long illness with breast cancer. Terry had already lost his sister in a fatal auto accident and his father had disappeared from his life soon after he was born. Diane was there to hold Terry at his mother's death. He seemed completely alone in the world, with no family member to care for him. Diane's grief was evident as she told how she advocated for Terry, creatively gathering together the resources of his community to find for him the support he needed to get him through the next weeks, months, and years. To her, more important than her superb technical skills or her expert performance in emergencies was the fact that she had been able to make a difference in the life of this one little boy. Through her story, I saw with the students how the expert nurse blends high-level technical skills with intuitive knowing to create the true art of nursing. It was a magical moment that I doubt any of us have ever forgotten, especially Diane.

Sharing stories between teacher and student, or student and client, is an example of the pedagogical thoughtfulness that can transform learning (Sorrell & Redmond 1997). Stories embody a personal way of knowing that is unique. As we listen to someone's story, we are drawn into the unique reality of that individual. This reality is often so personal and intimate that the stories may pour forth with unexpected tears from both storyteller and listener.

Case Studies and Narratives

When the faculty in the College of Nursing and Health Science at George Mason University (GMU) decided to implement a community-based curriculum, one component of this curriculum was the use of narratives, or stories, as a teaching strategy. A seminar was integrated into each clinical course to provide the students with experience in writing and telling stories about their clients and about their own personal experiences. Most faculty, however, were unfamiliar with the use of stories as a teaching strategy and some perceived it as "fluff" — "touchy, feeling" activities that had no sound basis in teaching and learning. As a result, the intended *stories* of clients' experiences sometimes evolved into *case studies*, which were more familiar to both faculty and students.

Case studies can serve as useful teaching and learning strategies, but they exemplify a different way of learning than do stories. To write a case study, a student usually goes to the client's medical record to gather facts about a diagnosis, demographics, lab values, or treatment regimens. Alternatively, students may take a case study from a text to analyze. The end result of either of these approaches is a structured presentation of facts from which the student may deduce a plan of care.

The use of stories involves a more inductive approach. The student goes to the client as the source, not the medical record or a text. Through stories, the student gathers data on the *meaning* of the illness experience to the client. This seems especially important when caring for clients in community-based settings, where clients may often be isolated from day-to-day contacts with health-care professionals and thus struggle to manage their health in the way that seems best to them.

The differences that these two teaching strategies can have in terms of student learning are illustrated by my experience with two students who were responsible for presenting content on incontinence to their classmates. One student used a traditional case study to present this information, providing details of her plan of care for an elderly woman who had been her patient in a nursing home. She did an excellent presentation of the physiological aspects of voiding and the different types of incontinence. She presented information about diagnostic tests and offered strategies for dealing with incontinence. Students were attentive and dutifully took notes on her presentation.

In contrast, a student in another class told a story of what it was like to care for her husband after he returned home from a prostatectomy (she had obtained his permission to tell his story). She told of her husband's concern at having to buy and wear incontinence pads under his elegant suits and his embarrassment with "accidents" that sometimes occurred at work. Her husband asked his physician how long the incontinence would last, and when the physician said "not long," her husband interpreted that to be a week, at the most. Therefore, when he was still leaking urine in the fourth week after surgery, he was panicky that this would be permanent. As this student told her story, there was intense stillness among the students and a palpable bond formed between storyteller and listeners. Students were moved by their new awareness of what it meant to live with this problem that before had seemed so trivial. Some students shared their own stories of problems

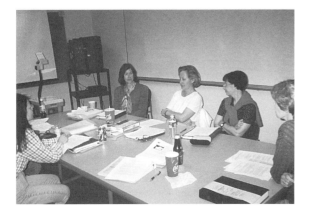

with incontinence. The physiological and psychological aspects of the problem came naturally into the discussion, so that the class learned this information as it applied to a specific person's problem. Students took fewer notes because they were so involved in the discussion. I would have loved to give a "post-test" to these two classes to see which class scored higher on content related to "problems with incontinence." However, I do not think the test would have been a true indicator of the learning that took place through the storytelling; the real learning was how it changed our personal understandings of what it might mean to live with this problem.

COMPOSITION RESEARCH

Research in composition during the past three decades has helped us to understand that not only is it important for students to learn to write, but also it is important for them to *use* writing to *learn*. Emig (1983) carried out research on the composing processes of high school students and concluded that in the process of writing, connections are made between the hand, eye, and brain that can lead to new insights and facilitate learning. Other researchers in composition have expanded our understanding of the thinking processes inherent in the practice of writing. Thus, we now know that the *process* of writing serves as a valuable tool for *learning*, as well as for communication (Thaiss 1991, Young 1997). It is important for faculty to view writing not only as a finished *product* with appropriate style, grammar, and spelling, but also as a *process* that can help students to make important connections between ideas.

Britton (1975) noted in his research that most writing that students do in the classroom is formal and scientific, a type of writing he termed *transactional*. A reliance on transactional writing shows limited understanding of how language relates to the thinking process. Britton noted the need for students to explore *expressive writing*, which is a type of writing often addressed to oneself or to a trusted person, such as in diaries, journals, letters, or first-draft papers. Expressive writing is the type of writing that is most personal and may be closest to the thinking process itself. Stories are one important form of expressive writing. Research has demonstrated that this type of writing is crucial for trying out and coming to terms with new ideas (Britton 1975, Thaiss 1991).

Thus, when students are assigned to write stories, these stories serve not only as a mode of communication, but as a form of learning in itself. This process of writing offers an important opportunity for students to connect ideas from internal and external sources, critically think about the ideas, and then infer a generalization that gives the separate pieces of information a coherent verbal shape.

Mary was an experienced RN who came back to school for her BSN and participated in a writing-intensive nursing class. Her comments illustrate how the use of writing as a teaching strategy is much more than a way to help students improve their writing; it is a way to help them come to understand.

A Student's Perspective

 Day One: I sat in the class unsettled. This feeling was not due to "course expectations." I had brought the unsettled, anxious feeling with me. I was experiencing what I had heard and read about too often in nursing—professional burnout. As a clinician with two decades of experience in the emergency setting, I was disillusioned in my practice. Perhaps it was all the restructuring, the aging process, my low endorphins, or an overdue midlife crisis. Whatever, it was happening, and I was ready to step out of my nursing role, throw out my beat-up tennis shoes, and simply move on. I was still searching, however, for the new direction I would take.

Mid-semester: As the semester proceeded, I began to realize subtle changes in my mood, as well as the perceptions of my classmates. The poignant writings found in the reservoir of untapped talent, buried in the hearts, minds, and souls of each student, started to surface. This wellspring of creativity and caring exposed a core of nursing I had never known before. The genuine humanism found in personal stories was stunning. I felt a sense of renewal and deep sense of pride for my profession.

Transition: I left this class more unsettled than when I arrived. At the beginning, I was doubtful that I would remain in nursing. Now I knew that I needed to advance my profession through my writing, but I wasn't sure how. I returned to my emergency nursing practice, wearing the same ragged Reeboks and juggling even more job demands than before. My direction is still uncertain but my purpose is clear. I have become painfully aware of the need for new words to strike down what is dreadful in our present health-care system and to lift up what has hope to be.

This class served as my launching pad for publication, giving me confidence to write about my profession. It helped me to polish my style and streamline my manuscripts. But, the most important lesson I learned in the class was a sense of responsibility. Now, in the midst of my hectic schedule, I take the necessary "time out," shut the door, and hang out my shingle which cautions: "Quiet, please, there is a nurse writing."

STRATEGIES FOR USING STORYTELLING IN TEACHING

Storytelling is often viewed as a feminist learning strategy, in that storytelling may come more naturally for women than for men (Sorrell 2001). Thus, it is interesting to think how this teaching strategy relates to male students. Patterson and colleagues (1995), in a phenomenological study with 20 male students in a baccalaureate nursing program, explored male nurses' perceptions of how they learned to care during their nursing education experiences. Both beginning and senior male students described the process of learning to care as enhanced by listening to and reflecting on stories, including stories from nurses, teachers, friends, and classmates. These students also stated that they sought out stories from nursing home residents in an attempt to understand the experience of being a patient.

Storytelling in the Nursing Classroom

The activity of storytelling may seem strange in a formal classroom where students are used to listening passively to a lecture or discussion. It is important to recognize that when storytelling is initiated as a teaching strategy in the classroom, it may create an unanticipated intimacy that initially may be uncomfortable for students. It is helpful to engage students in thinking about this before they read their stories aloud. It is important to create a safe learning environment in the classroom so that students feel secure in sharing their stories and disclosing personal feelings (Geanellos 1996).

The following is an example of what happened in one of my classrooms:

 It was the last class before semester break and the time I had set aside for reading stories aloud. I had participated in a similar activity when attending a writing workshop for teachers a year ago. At that session, we all sat in a circle and, one by one, read a story aloud that we had written. The stories were wonderful—some sad, some hilarious, but all were very personal. It was an empowering experience that I had wanted to offer to my students.

The whole experience had seemed so simple and natural then. Now, with my own students, I felt frighteningly alone and unsure of whether this would really work. The students' anxiety was evident as they arranged themselves in a circle and pulled from their notebooks the stories they had written. I outlined a few ground rules for the session and then asked if someone would start with their story. Complete silence. The silence continued. I tried to mask my own anxiety. Finally, one brave student said that she would start.

This student read her story aloud, and then another student followed. Gradually, as the reading of the stories continued, a palpable energy took hold of us all. At one point a student faltered, her voice breaking at the unexpected emotion that came forth as she read her story. She was unable to continue, but the student next to her intuitively sought nonverbal permission, reached over for the piece of paper, and finished reading the story. When the circling of the readings arrived at me, I began to read my story aloud. I could sense the surprise of the students. They had not expected me to participate in the reading. My heart was pounding. This sharing of my own thoughts with students through a medium as intimate as writing was not easy!

Through practice with this strategy of having students read their stories aloud in class, I have learned to trust the process. During one storytelling activity in class, a student became overwhelmed with emotion and suddenly left the classroom. Afterward, she apologized and confided that her sister had died barely three months earlier. When she had listened to her classmate's story of a patient's death, she was suddenly confronted with her own grief. As we talked about this experience, we also talked together about the losses in our lives, and I realized that this was indeed a pedagogical moment. After the storytelling activity, I also received e-mails from students in the class who told me that even though they had cried during the storytelling, they valued the experience deeply.

Storytelling in Community-based Clinical Experiences

In community-based clinical experiences, students are often not face-to-face with faculty for many of their clinical hours, and thus need to function fairly independently. As noted in this text, journals and clinical conferences can be very useful strategies for encouraging students to write or talk about their clinical experiences, so that faculty know better how to guide their learning. Students' stories in journals or clinical conferences can provide important clues for the type of guidance students may need.

One student, Nancy, told me of an experience that was traumatic for her whole clinical group. Although it is a fairly long narrative, I have included it here because I believe embedded in this story are many poignant facets of learning for which students need guidance:

It was our psych rotation, our second year, our last semester. We were in the clinical setting without having somebody there with us.... It was a woman's center and we all had to go there. We all sat down and watched these films, the first one was on alcoholism, which was really, really good. It was called "Chalk Talk."...And then they had a film on, it was very graphic... on children who were in an abuse situation, and they actually portrayed this family, this mother and father, and they were actually abusing the kids.... Probably over half the people in our class had been touched with the problems of alcoholism or abuse, whether it be by spouse or father. And for the first time, they're seeing, they're having to look at their childhood. You know, you were always on the inside with your little perspective on life. And then all of a sudden, you're on the outside looking in, saying, "Oh, my god, he was really a mess." And so instead of seeing those little kids, you're seeing your own self.

Afterward, we all sort of gathered outside before we left, and everyone was wandering around.... We were in shock. You know? We were like—We felt like we'd been bombed. And then, all of a sudden it was OK, we're professional now, we don't think about this anymore.... The person I carpool with, she's young, 19, and is still living right in the situation and for her it was very, very, very hard...she was really falling apart, she didn't know what to do with it. She was just, uncontrollably crying....

Later, we went to our faculty members, and even the head faculty member, I felt like she was patting us on the head, you know.... The response was, "well, you'll get over it." It was like shoved aside, that you have to learn about these problems, the mental illnesses, depression, anxiety, and the whole gamut of everything so that you can recognize it in other people, but it doesn't happen to you.

I wrote about it in my journal and sometimes they (faculty) would write in it, on the edge of the thing you know and say, well, "keep verbalizing," but it was just frustrating because at first I thought maybe they were doing it to screen out and realize that if someone's really having some problems, they could call them into their office... and let's make an avenue for it, but they never did....

At these clinicals, one instructor is in charge of all these different facilities, so you have to be there at eight in the morning, but she may not show up until like noon, and then she's there for an hour and then gone to go to another, that's like an hour away. So if you're going through something, I mean like the very first day, going to a place like that.... It's so overwhelming to see, you know 20 or 30 schizophrenic, depressed people just like wandering around, spaced out, and acting all kinds of weird ways, and.... you leave thinking maybe you're not so normal after all, and it's really a weird situation....

There were a lot of people, a lot of people who I know didn't even get to where I was and even cry about it. You know, you could see that they just sort of took a deep breath and said, "OK, I'm not going to think about this anymore." But if you don't deal with it as it comes every time, then how are you going to help somebody else? (Redmond & Sorrell, 1996).

Community-based clinical experiences impose unique pressures on both students and faculty. It is important for both to take time to listen to these stories.

STRATEGIES FOR EFFECTIVE TEACHING WITH STORIES

Most students probably have had much more experience in writing "research," or technical papers than stories. Therefore, when asked to write a story, they may be hesitant and unsure of how to proceed. They also need guidance in how to share their stories with others through reading them.

Composing an Effective Story

I find that a useful, and fun, way to ease into writing a story is to do a "madman" writing. I tell the students to think of a topic to write about in class and that they will have three minutes to write it. There are only two rules:

1. They must keep writing, not lifting their pens from the paper as they write. If they seem blocked and cannot think of how to continue the story, they can write "I feel blocked" and then try to continue writing;
2. They should not "censor" their writing by going back and crossing something out or correcting a misspelling. The focus should be on getting creative thoughts down on paper without worrying about the "shoulds" and the "should nots."

I time them during the exercise, telling them exactly when to start and stop. Afterward, we talk about what thoughts came out on paper and what parts of their writing would make good parts of a story. This exercise helps students to experience their own creative energies and to see how the free, unhindered writing can help them to form unexpected connections between ideas. Students are encouraged to set aside time at home, 5 to 10 minutes at a time, to begin another story and to write regularly. I emphasize that writing must be practiced. Like physical exercise, it is not enough just to read about it—it must be done!

I have found that students enjoy writing a group story and that this is a non-threatening way to help them see how a story can be written simply. I write the beginning of a "nurse mystery," sometimes about Cherry Ames, the fictitious nurse heroine of another generation. Many students do not know who Cherry Ames was and others enjoy explaining about her and how nursing has changed. Box 3–1 provides an example of one possible story beginning.

Box 3-1 | Learning Exercise for Faculty Use

Cherry Ames, RN: A Nurse Mystery at Fairfax Hospital

Cherry Ames, RN, hurried down the hall to Mr. Jones' room. This was her first day on the unit and she was feeling insecure. Mr. Jones had seemed very anxious when she met him the night before and even said that someone was trying to hurt him. The nurses told her that he was confused and hallucinating, yet he had no history of this prior to his hospitalization. At the entrance to Mr. Jones' room, Cherry stopped short in surprise.

I read the beginning of the story to the class and then pass it to a student in the front of the room. Each student writes one sentence that forwards the "plot" of the story and then passes it on to the next student. Meanwhile, I am teaching the class as I would any other time but can observe as the paper makes its way through the class. The students are momentarily distracted while writing their sentences but then quickly focus again on the lecture or discussion material being presented. At the end of the class period, I read the story aloud. Each student enjoys hearing her or his contribution, and some of the entries are hilarious! This exercise seems to help students see that there is nothing too simple to be accepted; after this often rambling and disconnected story, they know that their own efforts have to be better!

I give students specific guidelines for writing an effective story (Box 3–2). I also read them some stories that students in previous classes have written, and we discuss what makes the stories powerful. (I maintain the confidentiality of the authors of these stories and get their permission to read them.) They then write a draft of their story at home and bring a draft to class. We sometimes set aside time at the end of class to form small peer reading and writing groups to hear and critique the stories. I model for the students how to give constructive feedback on a classmate's writing. The author gains insight into what aspects of the story resonate with the listener and what parts may distract from the flow of the story. Students also learn an important skill in being able to critique the writing without offending the author.

Reading Stories in the Classroom

I plan two sessions during a semester for students to read their stories aloud. These are, for the students as well as me, powerful learning experiences. Students have worked their stories through several drafts until they are polished. The experience for students in the class to hear the author read her or his own personal story, and the experience for the author to see the reaction of the audience, creates important pedagogical understandings.

I call the storytelling activity a "Read Around." We sit in a circle, and I ask one student to volunteer to start. After this first story, there may be some brief comments, but we do not stop to analyze the story or discuss it in-depth. The focus is on the storytelling itself and the message it conveys, not the construction of it. The storytelling then moves onto the next volunteer until everyone has had an opportunity to read. If someone does not wish to read his or her story, I do not require it, but I do strongly encourage all students to participate, for I think it is a valuable experience for them. I inform them when they first write their story that we will be reading them in class and that they may not want to write about something so personal that they would not want to share it with others. During the Read Around, I also read a story to the class that I have written. Students often are surprised that I, too, read a story I have written, but I believe that they value my willingness to participate. I strongly believe that as faculty, if we want our students to experience the pleasure of writing, we must also do it ourselves.

Evaluating Students' Stories

Most writing assignments in nursing are designed to assess students' learning of the subject matter and require transactional or "scientific" writing, not expressive writing. Yet if students are to develop skills in inference so that they can put together pieces of information from their readings and experience to create new understandings and meanings, then they must be guided to go beyond the limits of transactional writing. Transactional writing promotes closure. In contrast, expressive writing is not as constrained by form and style and provides students with an opportunity to "play" and experiment with ideas and to value the thinking process itself. Students

---

Box 3-2   Learning Exercise for Faculty Use

Writing an Effective Story

Describe an incident related to health care that stands out in your mind because it went exceptionally well and made a real difference in your life.

Describe an incident that stands out in your mind because there was a frustrating breakdown in providing effective health care.

Describe an incident related to health care in which you made a mistake.

Describe an incident related to health care that was a special challenge.

Describe an incident that you think illustrates the essence of what nursing is about.

Try these guidelines for writing your story:

Write in the first person, using simple phrases, just as you would tell it to a friend. Include important details that help the reader understand the context, or background, in which the experience occurred. Be careful, though, not to include unnecessary details that distract the reader from the main story line. Describe why the incident is "critical." State what concerns, thoughts and feelings were occurring during the incident.

Stories are often only 1 to 2 pages. Think about how you want your story to begin and end. If you present too much background information, especially at the beginning, your readers may lose interest before they get to the main message of the story. Try to begin your story in an interesting way that makes the reader want to continue reading. Also, you want to end your story in a way that leaves the reader thinking about the message of this "never again" story.

Adapted from Brenner, 1984.

need opportunities to experiment with different writing styles, including writing for themselves, rather than for the professor.

This means that faculty need to think carefully about how they will evaluate students' stories. It is important to be clear on what you want the students to learn from the story writing. Evaluation criteria on such aspects as giving evidence to support a claim, the number and kinds of sources cited, and the number and accuracy of the specific facts given are not appropriate for evaluating expressive writing. Instead, they send a message to students that it is the scientific facts and deductive reasoning that are important, not the power of the individual experience. In many ways, learning through stories is inductive learning.

Students may feel self-conscious about using expressive writing and fear that they appear immature. Students need to see that faculty value this type of writing as a way to verbalize thoughts not yet well-defined, using language as a way to discover what they want to say. Self-awareness and self-knowledge are essential for thinking critically.

I believe that it is important to differentiate between *evaluating* students' written work and *grading* it. I often give the completed story a "checkmark," sometimes with a "plus" or "minus," instead of a letter grade. Sometimes I involve the students in helping me to devise evaluation criteria that they believe are meaningful. Because the stories often describe experiences that the students care about deeply, I find it difficult to award letter grades, which seem to stamp an "excellent," "good," or "average" label on a very personal experience. The students know that they need to write a polished story before they will receive credit for it and are allowed to do multiple drafts of the assignment, incorporating feedback from their peer reading and writing groups and from my review of the story. Because the stories are usually only 1 to 2 pages, I find that I can quickly read them and provide some suggestions for strengthening them.

Some nursing faculty may not feel confident in critiquing students' written stories. They may feel it is inappropriate for students to have "help" on a paper through drafts critiqued by peers or by faculty. We have found it helpful to form partnerships with faculty in the English department. Joint meetings between English and nursing faculty have enhanced nursing faculty's understanding and confidence in trying out new approaches for teaching students about writing. Faculty in the English department have offered workshops for nursing faculty to learn about current research and teaching methodologies in writing-intensive courses. An added benefit is that English faculty, through reading students' poignant stories, have come to see nursing in a new way.

Showcasing Students' Stories

Students are proud of the stories produced in their class and may want to "showcase" the stories in various ways (Sorrell 2001). One of these projects involved designing a desk calendar with a student's story for each month and additional stories and pictures interspersed throughout the calendar. When students gave these calendars to friends and families as gifts, they received many compliments about the positive image of nursing conveyed by the stories. Some of these calendars were centered around a theme for a nursing organization and sold as a fundraising activity.

Another project was the development of a Web site featuring students' stories, which they called "Weaving a Tapestry of Nursing Care through Stories" (Sorrell 2001). Students not only gained valuable writing skills through the project, but also learned the technical aspects of designing a Web site. The Web site was publicized at a University-wide "Innovations" conference. Students and faculty who read the stories on the Web site came away with a new understanding of the many parameters of nursing.

One of the most effective outcomes of story writing in my classes was a book, *Beveled Edges: A Portrait of Caring. Nurses' Reflections* (College of Nursing and Health Science 2000), published online. The title reflected students' perceptions of their stories as a valuable portrait protected in a bevel-edged frame. Students completed publication of the book in one semester by separating into work groups to focus on proposal writing, editing, graphics, and marketing. They obtained a grant of $160 from an online publisher to cover publication costs for 30 books. Students spent many hours editing their stories to ensure that they were free of grammatical errors and that they did not betray confidentiality of patients described in the stories. Students obtained photographs to illustrate the various stories, scanned them, and sent them to the online publisher. The project was publicized in the campus newspaper and other sources, and students identified feasible options for selling the book. They decided to pay $7 for each of their own books so that the 30 free books could be used as samples to distribute to bookstores for sale. Students took pride in knowing that all proceeds from book sales went to a scholarship fund.

This project seemed to take on a life of its own as students lingered after class to discuss progress with their book. Through participation in the project, students gained not only oral and written communication skills, but also skills in editing, marketing, scanning graphics, and collaborating. Students' engagement with the project was evidenced through their continued e-mail dialogues after the class ended, in which they shared more stories of enthusiastic comments they received from purchasers of the book. The archivist for the University requested a copy of the book, the Dean of the College sent some to the University Board of Visitors, and students, faculty, and persons outside the University purchased other copies. Students' pride in the project is illustrated by one student's description of a humorous experience: While attending a meeting in her clinical agency, a nurse passed around the *Beveled Edges* book and asked her, "Have you seen this book?" "Seen it?" the student responded with great satisfaction, "I helped to write it!" (Sorrell 2001).

In closing this chapter, I would like to include a final story—one that I wrote and read aloud to students during our Read Around for the last class of the semester and which I included in the *Beveled Edges* book (College of Nursing and Health Science 2000). I hope it helps to convey the power that came from sharing our stories together in our classroom throughout the semester.

> Although many of your paradigms this semester were about patients, I had no patients to care for. My responsibilities as a nurse educator and administrator increasingly limit my contact with patients, and I deeply miss the clinical world that used to be such an important part of my life. Sometimes I envy you as I listen to your stories of patients you cared for, knowing you made a difference in their lives.
>
> In a sense, you are my patients now, for as I interact with you, I reap many of the same kinds of rewards I got from caring for patients. When I think back to the first day of our class together, I remember how cold and impersonal our classroom felt—just four walls, full of empty chairs facing straight ahead. But as the semester progressed, that cold classroom seemed to become energized at 4:30 on Tuesdays. Little changes occurred. I was nervous in the beginning about assigning you a nonmedical story to read, "Average Waves in Unprotected Waters," afraid you would think this was some sort of wifty class. But your discussion of this story was sensitive, probing, and beautiful. I began to sense that we had a very special class, and as the semester evolved, I came to realize the amazing talent that filled our nursing classroom each Tuesday. Food began to arrive magically each week— wonderful food—lugged into the classroom from distant parking lots. Breaks became longer and livelier as we came to know each other.
>
> There never seemed to be enough time in our class period! As a teacher, I look back over the semester and the topics we discussed and wish I had more time to "cover" things. There is so much more I want to discuss. But then I remember the advice of one of my teachers, who said that "to cover" is to cover over, to hide, and that as teachers and students, we should be concerned not about covering content, but about uncovering it, about bringing forth and lighting up new ideas and insights.
>
> If our classroom could talk, I think it would have many stories to tell. In the process of our meeting each week to discuss a specific topic, many other things have happened in our lives. Some of us experienced profound losses—losses involving a family member, friend, or patient. These lives can never be recovered. They change us forever as we try to integrate the loss into our being. Patricia Benner (1984) says that we're changed by nursing interactions, and I've been changed through interacting with you this semester. Together we've uncovered new ways of knowing about nursing. Even with topics such as wound healing, anxiety, incontinence, nausea, and pain, we learned to apply art, music, and poetry to nursing. We've laughed together, and we've cried. I've seen you reach out to support each other through the stress of presenting your seminars and writing your papers and paradigms, and you have supported me. Through these past months, I saw us gradually grow as a community of nurse scholars, caring nurse scholars. In some ways, I feel a loss at the semester's end, knowing that our classroom will once more be cold and silent on Tuesdays at 4:30. But the classroom will find new stories to tell. I know that your special stories need to expand beyond the classroom—to our patients, loved ones, and to all nurses—a finely chiseled portrait of caring (College of Nursing and Health Science 2000).

References

Benner, P (1984). From novice to expert: Excellence and power in clinical nursing practice. Menlo Park, CA: Addison Wesley.

Britton, J (1975). The development of writing abilities 11-18. London: MacMillan.

College of Nursing and Health Science (2000). Beveled edges: A portrait of caring. Nurses' reflections. Fairfax, VA: George Mason University. Produced by Chapbooks: www.chapbooks.com.

Emig, JA (1983). The web of meaning. Upper Montclair, NJ: Boynton/Cook.

Geanellos, R (1996). Storytelling: A teaching-learning technique. Contemp Nurse 5(1), 28-35.

Patterson, B L, et al. (1995). How male nursing students learn to care. J Adv Nurs 22(3), 600-609.

Redmond, GM & Sorrell, JM (1996). Voices of Caring: The lived experience of nursing students. Unpublished research.

Sorrell, JM (2001). Stories in the nursing classroom: Writing and learning through stories. Language and Learning Across the Discipline. (in press).

Sorrell, JM, & Redmond, GM (1997). The lived experiences of students in nursing: Voices of caring speak of the tact of teaching. J Prof Nurs 13(4), 228-235.

Thaiss, CJ (1991). Write to the limit. Fort Worth: Holt, Rinehart, and Winston.

Van Manen, M (1991). The tact of teaching. Albany, NY: State University of New York.

CHAPTER 4

Teaching and Learning Activities in Community-based Settings

Georgine M. Redmond

Learning Objectives

1) Discuss three teaching or learning strategies used in community-based settings: journaling, postconference, and learning portfolios.

2) Explore the concept of reflection involved in these teaching or learning strategies.

3) Describe the appropriate learning environment in which reflection occurs.

The community-based curriculum prepares students for current nursing practice and for the changes to come in the new millennium. Since 1986 (Tanner 1990), nurse educators have discussed a major paradigm shift in nursing education that was referred to as a curriculum revolution. Preparing nurses in this new paradigm as empowered, emancipated, and caring (Hays 1994) was the goal of nursing education. Learning experiences in this new paradigm would "… emphasize connectedness over separation, understanding over assessment, collaboration over debate, that allow time for knowledge to emerge from firsthand experiences, and encourage students to evolve their own patterns of work…." (Murray 1989, pp 198–199). Leaders in this new movement encouraged nurse educators to question the assumptions that undergird the selection of teaching and learning activities, focusing on not only what was taught but how it was taught.

More recently the American Association of Colleges of Nursing (AACN) published *The Essentials of Baccalaureate Education* (1998). The importance of active learning strategies to engage students in their own learning was stressed. Hays (1994) suggests that the "criteria for selecting learning activities include requirements that the activities be reality based and that they lead to insights, engagement with the concepts, dialogue, inquiry, and meaning making" (p 151). Bartels (1999) states that faculty have a responsibility in building a learning community and must "develop new ways to teach the growing amounts of knowledge and skills required of new graduates, develop innovative means to provide this knowledge and experience in diverse and often unique settings, use active learning strategies and real-life experiences and use an integrated approach to teaching across the curriculum."

Hays (1994) notes that these learning strategies can be developed and implemented more easily in the community.

In this chapter I will discuss three learning activities: journaling, postconference, and learning portfolios that can be used with students in community-based sites. These activities, when used appropriately, can help students actively engage in and make meaning from their learning experiences.

REFLECTION

First, let me discuss a key element in all of these learn-ing activities: reflection.

According to Pierson (1998), there are different understandings of the meaning of the phenomenon of reflection. Pierson believes that the significance of reflection in nursing education has come from the need to encourage students to think critically and to be innovative. As she says, "reflection in these new curricula is often considered the appropriate vehicle for the analysis of nursing practice, fostering not only an understanding of nurses' work, but also the development of the critically thoughtful approaches essential for providing nursing care in complex environments" (p 2). Pierson believes that reflection is both a technique and a process. This involves a combination of calculative thinking "...an abstract and practical process confined to organizing, managing and controlling" (p 2), and contemplative thinking, "...a natural and spontaneous process fundamental to the exploration of meaning" (p 2). She believes that nursing students begin reflective practice with calculative thinking and that time is necessary for them to think through the individual occurrences in their nursing practice and consider reasons for their thought, feeling, and actions about the event. Students can be encouraged to reflect both in writing and orally.

Trust is an important element in reflection if faculty intend to dialogue with students regarding their thoughts and feelings. The relationship between the faculty and student must be built on mutual respect and trust. Whether the reflection occurs in writing or orally, students must feel comfortable in sharing thoughts, feelings, and beliefs. Often this trust is built over time as the faculty-student relationship develops. Faculty must respond to students' reflection in sensitive and compassionate ways. Understanding perspectives and coming to terms with the meaning of the learning experience shared is a process that occurs in a trusting environment that faculty must create.

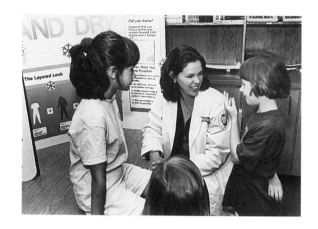

Journaling

According to Mayo (1996), "Journaling is a new paradigm teaching/learning technique. It can be operationalized so that students report, reflect, and analyze their experience" (p 27). As educators seek ways to help students reflect, journals provide one opportunity to do that. Journals can be used to strengthen students' calculative thinking as they record specific patient data like lab values and medications. As mentioned earlier, this may be the first step to reflective journaling. Others see journals as an opportunity to "think aloud" and record perceptions about clinical experiences (Brown & Sorrell 1993). Students have the opportunity to reflect on the experience in their journal and to see what they have learned from that experience. According to Sorrell and colleagues (1997), "The process of writing offers an opportunity for students to connect ideas from internal and external sources, critically think about ideas, and then infer a generalization that gives the separate pieces of information a coherent verbal shape" (p14). Kielinen (1997) used reflective journaling in a bridge program to give students the opportunity to reflect in a written form on activities and topics that were discussed. Students were encouraged to "...reflect on how they 'connected' and not simply record an event or discussion that occurred" (p 8). To build trust, students were told that the only person who would read their journal was their faculty member, that journals were ungraded, and that there was no "right" or "wrong" way to approach journaling. In addition, students were told that if there was a desire to use their journal comments, it would be with their permission and without names used. Part of the way the journaling was introduced in this program allowed students to listen to journal comments made by another class. This helped to broaden their perspectives and to give them a model. Most authors do not believe that journaling should be used as an assessment tool, (Brown & Sorrell 1993, Kielinen 1997, Pierson 1998) but instead to provide opportunities for dialogue with and thoughtful feedback from faculty.

Journals may be kept on a daily basis and collected weekly. Students should be given some structure as to the content and process suggested in their journal. Guidance may be given as to length of an individual entry as well. You may wish to ask students to describe their most meaningful event that day or ask them to discuss how a particular concept or objective was met. It is also important to ask the student to reflect on the impact the experience had on them personally or on their nursing practice.

Brown and Sorrell (1993) suggest three guidelines for clinical journals:

1. Identify outcomes for using the journal and give clear directions for assignments. Clinical journals may be used to document observations of patients, critique data according to relevant theories, suggest hypotheses and evaluate them, and write a critique.
2. Provide clear guidelines for journal entries, such as having students write their own learning objectives and how they are meeting them; write a summary of a clinical event or an article relevant to their current clinical experience; and write a focused argument on a professional issue.
3. Provide thoughtful and immediate feedback to students to develop a dialogue between teacher and student (pp 16–18). Table 4–1 provides some useful guidelines for clinical journals in community-based settings.

Research in Journaling

Fonteyn and Cahill (1998) examined the effectiveness of using reflective clinical logs to improve students' thinking strategies and metacognition (cognitive awareness). According to Fonteyn and Cahill (p 1), "metacognition is often equated with critical thinking." Nine junior students in a baccalaureate nursing program participated in

---

Table 4-1

Guidelines for Clinical Journals in Community-based Settings

OBJECTIVES

1. Apply scientific data to community-based practice.
2. Encourage expression of thoughts, feelings, and attitudes about clinical experiences.
3. Expand personal and professional perspectives.
4. Increase critical-thinking skills.

GUIDELINES FOR JOURNAL

1. Write daily learning objectives, and date each entry.
2. Write descriptive observations of clinical events.
3. Discuss challenges and conflicts experienced.
4. Discuss feelings, perceptions, and reactions about the day's events.
5. Discuss any community-based concepts that you applied—for instance, health, communication, prevention, or interdisciplinary teams.
6. Journals should be two to three pages in length.

HELPFUL HINTS

1. Write your entry as close to the events as possible.
2. Try to develop your thoughts fully.
3. Remember—don't just record an event: reflect on the experience with personal viewpoints and theoretical connections.

JOURNALS ARE REQUIRED BUT NOT GRADED.

JOURNALS WILL BE READ ONLY BY YOUR CLINICAL FACULTY AND NOT SHARED WITHOUT YOUR PERMISSION.

the study. Students did not develop nursing care plans for their patients but instead used an inductive approach through reflection in their clinical logs. These students wrote in detail about the patients and other clinical data. At the end of the week the faculty wrote on the thinking strategies that the students had used in their journals. For example, recognizing patterns, forming relationships, generating hypotheses, providing explanations and having conclusions were possible thinking strategies used. The students preferred the logs to nursing care plans because they felt the logs helped them to improve their ability to think about their thinking. Faculty found that students demonstrated those thinking strategies used by practicing nurses. According to Fonteyn and Cahill, "Clinical logs provide a means for faculty to assist students to identify, refine and develop the critical cognitive skills that they will use in their practice" (p 6).

In another study, Sorrell and colleagues (1997) investigated using portfolio assessment to document critical-thinking outcomes in nursing students. Researchers found that clinical logs were best representative of critical thinking in student portfolios. In these logs students demonstrated that they could translate technical nursing language and express unique perspectives on their experiences to nonnursing audiences.

The following are some excerpts from reflective journals that address the problem of violence in society.

VIOLENCE IN MUSIC

In order to hear an account of violence in music lyrics, I had to search beyond the CDs, tapes, and radio stations I listen to. I am a big fan of country music and there really isn't a great amount of violence noted in those kind of songs. While I was visiting a friend this past week, I remembered about this assignment and asked if I could look at his music selections. I came across a song by the group Nine Inch Nails titled "Big Man with a Gun." Here were some of the lyrics: "I am a big man (yes I am) and I have a big gun; got me a big old . . . and I like to have fun: held against your forehead, . . . maybe I'll put a hole in your head; you know, just for the f___ of it.... I'm every inch a man, and I'll show you somehow; me and my f___ing gun; nothing can stop me now; shoot shoot shoot shoot...."

I was absolutely shocked after sitting down to really listen to those lyrics. With those kinds of songs, it is very hard to understand the words but with the help of my friend, we figured it out.

What an amazing message! I was speechless. It seems that rock music lyrics have become increasingly explicit—particularly with reference to drugs, sex, violence, and of even greater concern, sexual violence.

These songs and others like them contain some of the most disgusting thoughts I've ever heard, but they are more than just offensive. When combined with all the violence depicted by the whole range of media, they are helping to create a culture of violence that is increasingly enveloping our children and desensitizing them to consequences.

In order to help this problem, I believe that performers (in this case the music group Nine Inch Nails) need to take on the responsibility to serve as positive role models for children and teenagers. By producing lyrics like the ones above, they are doing quite the opposite. And again, I think that parents need to take a more active role in monitoring the music their children are exposed to and what they purchase.

Another account of violence I came across in music lyrics was in a song by Motley Crue called "Girls, Girls, Girls." The lyrics went something like this: "the blade o my knife, faced away from your heart; those last few nights, it turned and sliced you apart; laid out cold, now we're both alone, but killing you helped me keep you home." Again, another amazing and shocking account of graphic violence and suicide in music.

There really are no words to describe how disturbing this is to me. In the past, I have never really paid attention to the exact words of songs and now that I have I am sad. Sad that our society allows for this kind of stuff to disperse throughout our younger children and teenagers. I was reading somewhere that children today spend an average of approximately four to six hours a day listening to music either on the radio or on MTV. This is a scary statistic if you think about the developmental stages that children and teens go through. Most are in a stage of identity vs. confusion looking for attention and understanding. And unlike parents, music and its messages offer an always available unqualified acceptance of these young children and teens. Many of the songs also seem to offer simple answers to complex problems, like the lyrics to the song above. It seems to maybe give children a source of authority for what they feel and do. This needs to stop!

I never realized how graphic some of the lyrics in the music industry are today. I don't know what, but something must be done to regulate the type of music allowed in the hands of Americans, especially in our young children.

OBSERVATION IN A LOCAL STORE

It was 5 p.m. on a Thursday afternoon when I observed a mother who was approximately in her mid-30s pushing a stroller with her son in it. Her son was approximately 2 years old and her daughter walking beside them was approximately 4 years old. The family was dressed in casual brand-name clothing and had a tidy appearance. As the family stepped on the escalator, the 4-year-old walked ahead followed by the stroller and mother. I heard the mother tell the little girl to sit down on the escalator step. The little girl ignored her and continued to stare aimlessly straight ahead. By the third warning the mother threatened to hit her daughter if she did not comply with her request. As the escalator descended to the intended floor, the little girl stepped off the step followed by her family. The mother suddenly yanked the little girl by the arm and pulled her aside. She began to grasp the little girl by the arms and using both hands began to shake her in defiance while scolding her. The little girl began to cry. The mother stood and began to walk away with the stroller as she hurriedly told the crying little girl to follow her. The look of annoyance was still prevalent in her face.

I think the whole situation could have been avoided had the daughter obeyed her mother's wishes. Unfortunately this did not occur and the little girl was punished. In a better handling of the situation, the mother should have rented a stroller in the mall that occupied two children, left one or both children at home with someone, or used the elevator to go down one floor. The mother was probably tired of bringing the children from one place to another and was angered by her daughter's defiance. The mother could have taken her aside and quietly told her that the behavior she was exhibiting was not appropriate and that the next time the incident was repeated, she would be punished. Shaking the daughter was inappropriate. Had this been a much younger child, the mother would have caused serious harm to the little girl. I was torn at the time and still am as to whether or not I should have approached the family and mentioned something. Somehow I felt I had no right since there was no "real" harm committed. However, the potential for serious harm was present. When I look back at the situation, I now feel that maybe I should have intervened.

K-MART SATURDAY AFTERNOON

A mother in her mid-30s, white, thin, clean, and pretty with her hair up in a ponytail, is looking down the aisles yelling, "Jason! Jason!" She is carrying a shopping basket filled with cleaning products. She is wearing running pants and a sweatshirt.

She spots the boy in the toy section (where I happen to be). Jason is about 5 years old. He is clean, sandy haired, and dressed in jeans, sneakers and a denim jacket. He is playing with some sort of action hero figure.

Mom heads down the aisle, full force.

Jason holds the toy out to his mother and asks, "Mom! Can I get this?"

"I have been looking all over for you!" She says, exasperated.

"But mom, can I...?"

She tears the toy from his hands and shoves it back onto the shelf.

"Come on." She pulls him by the jacket, "Let's go."

"You never let me get anything!" Jason sulks and walks slowly.

"Come on!" She says again and pushes him forward.

It looked to me as if the Mom was getting supplies maybe for weekend cleaning (not a fun job). She seemed to be in a hurry to pick up the items and go. She may have been scared when she couldn't find her son right away, then vented her fear and frustration on him. Kids, of course, will go to the TOY SECTIONS! Kids, like adults, see, like, and want. Naturally.

The way my mom always handled that sort of trip was to tell us BEFORE we went into the store that we were there to pick up XYZ only, not to shop for toys and did we think we could help her find those things? We were involved in a "scavenger hunt" and she knew where we were. I think you also have to accept the fact that things just may take a little longer if you're going to take children with you.

It was also not necessary to tear the toy from the child's hands and push him. He's only doing what kids will do. There are better ways to say "No" or "I was scared when I couldn't find you." Limits can be set gently.

Violence was done to this child both physically by pushing and rough handling, and emotionally as well by making him feel like he's "bad" because his mother lost track of him. What you want doesn't matter— that was the message I got.

A SUPPOSEDLY ROMANTIC MOVIE

"The Story of Us," a Rob Reiner film, starring Bruce Willis and Michelle Pfeiffer.

"Romantic!"

"The Most Romantic movie of the year!"

If that's true, it's a sad, sad year for romance.

This couple bickers, picks, nags, and blows up at each other for 90 of the longest minutes of movie history. They dutifully attempt a united front for their two children (how one does that while screaming in the house I don't know). They slam doors, throw things, hurl insults at one another, whine that the other isn't listening, accuse, and complain about their roles in the marriage. They consult with their shallow vulgar friends whose relationships are even more dilapidated than their own—minus the screaming.

In the end, I needed a TUMS, and they tearfully decided to stay together... all those "good times" they've had creating a warm fuzzy history worth "fighting for"... ironically.

What did I miss?

If this is a portrayal of a "normal" marriage, I sure am glad I'm single, and hope to stay that way happily ever after! Shame on Hollywood for turning a dysfunctional relationship into a romance! People who love each other do not scream and yell at each other. They do not insult and bicker constantly, and they do not decide that that's OK!

If we can accept violence in our closest of relationships, we can accept it on a much broader scale. If we accept this as "normal," as something "all couples go through," it's a sad, sad commentary on love and romance.

I didn't like the movie— it made me feel sad.

These reflective journal entries assist students to develop a sensitivity to the problem of violence in our society. Focusing on, recording, analyzing, and reflecting upon specific violent situations profoundly affects their willingness to become involved in all levels of violence prevention.

POSTCONFERENCES

Clinical postconference is an integral part of the clinical hours that students spend in practicum experiences. Letizia and Jennrich (1998) point out that little empirical evidence supports the educational benefits of such an experience. Oermann and Gaberson (1998) discuss using postconference for assessment purposes. Pierson

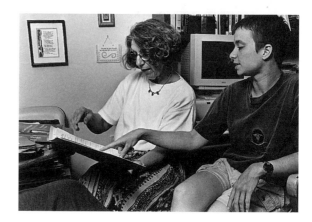

suggests using "clinical debriefing" (p 4) throughout the day to support students' reflections as they care for patients.

I would propose that using clinical postconference in community-based settings as an opportunity for reflection and to help students make meaning out of the day's events is yet another way to enhance critical thinking and help students to connect their experiences. Postconferences provide an opportunity not only for immediate instructor feedback but for feedback from peers as well.

In community-based settings faculty often have several groups of students in different agencies. It is essential that students and faculty meet daily for postconference to share and integrate the day's experiences. In a study on caring, Redmond and Sorrell (1996) found that when faculty were not on-site with students each day, the students described their experience as uncaring and sometimes even traumatic. Postconference is one way that faculty can keep students connected and supported.

Postconferences can provide a planned opportunity for clinical debriefing. Students have the opportunity to think through and discuss their experiences, as well as listen and learn from their colleagues. This type of postconference, unlike a structured classroom experience, is frequently driven by the group process of the students both in content selection and pace. The discussion allows students to revisit the day's experience and arrive at a new perspective.

> **Box 4-1** Learning Exercise for Faculty Use
>
> ## Postconference Reflection Questions
>
> Describe a situation that occurred today that was particularly frustrating or satisfying.
>
> ### Follow-up Questions
>
> - How did you feel about it?
>
> - How did you react?
>
> - Were other health-care providers involved?
>
> - Did you feel challenged? Why?
>
> - Was there any conflict in the situation? Describe it.

Research Related to Postconferences

The learning environment in postconference must be open and non-threatening. Letizia and Jennrich (1996) developed a Clinical Post-Conference Learning Environment Survey (CPCLES). The elements of the CPCLES were involvement, cohesion, teacher support, task orientation, order and organization, and innovation. They conducted a study to assess the psychometric properties of the tool as well as to explore and describe undergraduate student and faculty perceptions of clinical postconference learning environments. Sixty-four to 100 percent of faculty and students in 3 baccalaureate programs participated in the study. Research findings indicated that one of the six sub-scales—innovation—was perceived as happening least and having the least importance in the learning environment. However, both students and faculty perceived teacher support as occurring most frequently and having the most importance in the learning environment. The impact of the learning environment on the learning process and outcomes is an important consideration for nurse educators particularly as students are encouraged to reflect and take risks. Gonda (1990) studied the perceptions of learning environments in postconferences for associate-degree and baccalaureate students. Associate-degree students wanted more attention to relationship dimensions like teacher-student and student-student relationships as well as more task-oriented, rule-oriented conferences. Baccalaureate students wanted more peer interaction and more innovations in teaching and learning strategies.

Oermann and Gaberson (1998) suggest that postconference discussions can not only improve students' communication skills but also promote problem solving, decision making and critical-thinking skills as well. For this to occur, however, teachers must use higher level questions in postconference that focus on application, analysis, synthesis, and evaluation. Research suggests teachers do not use higher level questions with students. In a recent study on questioning as a teaching strategy, Sellappah and colleagues (1998) found 26 clinical teachers at 2 postconferences used predominantly low level questions. Neither teaching qualifications nor experience made a significant difference in these results.

Oermann and Gaberson (1998) suggest that questions used to evaluate critical thinking may be used to guide discussions in conferences. These are

- the purposes and goals to be met
- questions, issues, and problems to be resolved

- information and evidence on which they are basing their thinking
- concepts and theories applicable to the question, issue, or problem being discussed
- inferences and conclusions possible
- implications and consequences of their reasoning (p 127).

Postconferences are an effective teaching-learning method when the learning environment is supportive and faculty use higher-level questions to support students' cognitive functioning.

Learning Portfolios

Student learning portfolios (Table 4–2) can be a very effective teaching-learning tool in community-based settings. For the purpose of this chapter, a portfolio is defined as "a selection of assignments that a student has consciously assembled from a number of pieces produced over a semester or some other period of time" (Crouch & Fontaine 1994, p 306). In community-based settings, a learning portfolio can help the faculty to validate community competencies because faculty are often supervising students in multiple community sites. In our program, students' portfolios are helpful to senior public health faculty because they can see the community competencies and experiences that students had in their junior community-based practicum and build upon them. There are generally two types of student portfolios—"best works" and "growth and learning portfolios" (Oermann & Gaberson 1998). In our program these types are combined. Students begin with a growth and learning portfolio that they add to each semester (Table 4–3). During the capstone seminar in their last semester, they can select from all of the evidence in their portfolios to develop a "best works" portfolio. The best works portfolio is used to validate program outcomes like critical thinking and communication. This portfolio can also be used by the students in job interviews or to serve as a basis for professional development as they move through their careers. We encourage students to set professional goals for their first year of nursing practice and to continue to add to their portfolios.

Some type of reflective writing is an essential component of portfolio development as well. This type of writing will help students to develop perspectives on their learning that occurred in an experience, course, clinical, or even throughout the whole program of study. In a "growth and learning" portfolio, the reflective essay might be on the students' first clinical experiences. In a "best works" portfolio, the reflection might be on why the evidence is best works. Oermann and Gaberson (1998) identify three steps necessary for setting up a portfolio system:

> Step 1: Identify the purposes of the portfolio. These decisions are made regarding use of the portfolio for growth and learning, best works, or both. In addition,

---

Table 4-2

Student Learning Portfolios

Definition: "A portfolio is a collection and interpretation of your work that allows a teacher, employer, or other person to evaluate your abilities" (Annis & Jones 1995, p 185).

OBJECTIVE

1. Provide evidence of student's ability to meet programmatic outcomes.
   A. Provider of care
   B. Designer, manager, and coordinator of care
   C. Member of the profession

2. Demonstrate development of professional values and behaviors through providing evidence of work completed throughout the nursing program.

3. Develop a "best work" portfolio at the conclusion of the nursing program to evaluate program outcomes and to use for ongoing professional development.

EXAMPLE OF EVIDENCE

Papers, skill sheets, professional insights from clinical, or examples of written assessments, such as health, family, community, teaching plans/projects, care studies, pictures of posters, or evidence of honors and awards.

Each course will require elements of the portfolio. Students should feel free to include examples of other work.

Table 4-3

First-semester Junior-year Portfolio Guidelines

1. Personal essay reflecting on:

   A. What is nursing?

   B. What does it mean to be a professional nurse? Collected in NURS 333 for traditional students. Pictures of Nursing Project in NURS 334 for RNs and LPNs.

2. Academic chronology to include:

   A. Past accomplishments: awards received, volunteer activities, including professional organizations like ANA/VNA, specialty groups and SNA, community service, previous degrees, and experience (NURS 333 and NURS 334).

3. Professional insights from NURS 331 clinical experience.

Table 4-4

Possible Portfolio Content

- Clinical journals
- Short papers
- Term papers
- Process recordings
- Group reports
- Health-promotion projects
- Reflection papers on nursing
- Products associated with demonstrating clinical competencies (videos and competency sheets)
- Independent-study projects
- Class exercises
- Research projects
- Photos of classwork produced
- Newspaper or magazine articles that document achievement
- Programs from events in which you participated
- Job evaluations from current employment
- Teacher evaluation
- Letters of commendation, thanks, awards, or honors

faculty must decide whether data will be used for formative, summative, or both types of evaluation. The authors also suggest that decisions be made regarding whether portfolios will be used for clinical or course evaluation or for programmatic needs such as curriculum and program evaluation. Some portfolios are used for assessing prior learning for advanced placement purposes, so this needs to be determined as well. Faculty must also decide whether students will have input into the process and content of the portfolio.

Step 2: Identify the type of content to be included in the portfolio. Content included in the portfolio depends on the objectives and purpose of the portfolio. Table 4–4 gives a range of possibilities for evidence that may be included in a portfolio.

Another consideration requiring a faculty decision in this area is whether students are free to select the evidence to meet the objectives or if faculty will require the same material of all students. A combination of required materials and student-selected evidence usually works best. Faculty also need to define a minimum number of entries for a satisfactory portfolio. Faculty should also be available to discuss portfolio development with students. Annis and Jones (1995) recommend students be given a systematic method of presentation when the portfolio assignment is given. They note their experience shows that students need faculty assistance to understand the purpose of "reflective essays."

Step 3: Decide on the evaluation of the portfolio entries including criteria for evaluation of individual entries and the portfolio as a whole. Faculty must decide if the portfolio will be a graded requirement of a course or clinical. If the portfolio is to be graded, then evaluation criteria will need to be developed for individual assignments and the entire portfolio. In our program, because students are required to include some specific types of evidence from their coursework, evaluation criteria for those assignments are already reflected in the course syllabus. The portfolio itself is ungraded throughout the program. The "best works" portfolio receives a grade in the capstone seminar course (Table 4–5).

Table 4–5 Portfolio Evaluation

Your portfolio can potentially earn 50 points. These points are allocated as follows:

Organization (15 points)

    Clear statement of goals 1 2 3 4 5
    Introductory statement, which links portfolio to student
        goals and summary 1 2 3 4 5
    Table of Contents 1 2 3 4 5
                                                                       Total ____

Content (15 points)

    Items selected for inclusion 1 2 3 4 5
    Examples support core competencies and skills 1 2 3 4 5
    Examples effectively support professional values 1 2 3 4 5
                                                                       Total ____

Presentation (10 points)

    Items included are well written 1 2 3 4 5
    Appearance is professional 1 2 3 4 5
                                                                       Total ____

Overall Effect (10 points)

    Reflects entry competencies and skills 1 2 3 4 5
    Impact on faculty evaluators 1 2 3 4 5
                                                                       Total ____

(Adapted from Annis, L., and Jones, C. (1995): Student Portfolios: Their Objectives, Development and Use. In Seldin, P., and Associates (eds): Improving College Teaching. Bolton, MA: Anhen, pp 181–190.)

Portfolio criteria reflected above may be used in any course. Another consideration in the evaluation of the portfolio is whether the student has input into the evaluation of the portfolio through self-assessment.

Often student portfolios are used in courses and programs in which faculty develop teaching portfolios. Student learning may be improved if faculty share their portfolios with students. This helps them to understand how to select and sequence material. Faculty have always had access to student portfolios, but the reverse has not always been true. Cambridge (1996) believes that this type of sharing may result in better teaching and learning. Annis and Jones (1995) believe that the main difference between faculty and student portfolios is whether you are "approaching the teaching/learning process from the top-down perspective of the instructor or from the bottom-up view of the student" (p 182). Both portfolios arise from a need to document accomplishments. "Preparing a portfolio contributes to reflection on one's efforts and identification of areas for improvement. It also empowers the people preparing it to judge their own performance" (p 180). Crouch and Fontaine (1994) believe that no matter how portfolios are used in your program, they have valuable and important consequences for faculty and students. These include:

- Instructors get a better sense of what is working and what is not working in the classroom. Because pieces are not judged summatively until the end of the semester, both students and instructor can discuss assignments as trials for a final product.
- In programmatic use of portfolios, instructors collaboratively design the evaluation rubric and learn from one another's practices, thereby enhancing both teaching and learning.
- Students learn that they cannot expect everything they produce to be of equal quality, but that they have time to bring pieces up to some standard. They also learn how to judge their own work and develop their own standards, rather than waiting for someone to impose standards on them.
- If students choose a limited number of pieces for the portfolio, they also learn they can abandon work that they are not interested in or that is not—and may never be—successful.
- Students have the opportunity to show what they have learned about writing, not simply what they have learned for a midterm or final exam.
- Students have the pleasure of putting together something truly "finished for a course because they have time to do so" (p 327).

This chapter has discussed three teaching-learning activities that can easily be incorporated into your teaching in community-based sites. Journals and portfolios rely heavily on "writing to learn" (Sorrell et al. 1997, p 14). Postconferences give students an opportunity to improve communication skills and clinically debrief their experiences. Used appropriately, all activities include reflection and can improve problem solving, decision making and critical thinking.

References

American Association of Colleges of Nursing (1998). Essentials of baccalaureate education. Washington, DC: American Association of Colleges of Nursing.

Annis, L, & Jones, C (1995). Student portfolios: Their objectives, development and use. In P Seldin & associates (Eds). Improving college teaching (pp 181-190). Bolton, MA: Anhen.

Bartels, J (August 1999). Building a learning community. Paper presented at a faculty retreat of George Mason University College of Nursing and Health Science, Landsdowne, Loudon, VA.

Brown, HN, & Sorrell, JM (1993). Use of clinical journals to enhance critical thinking. Nurs Educ 18(5), 16-19.

Cambridge, BL (1996). The paradigm shifts: Examining quality of teaching through assessment of student learning. Innovative Higher Education 20(4), 287-297.

Crouch, MK & Fontaine, SI (1994). Student portfolios as an assessment tool. In DF Halpern & associates (Eds). Changing college classrooms (Ch. 17). San Francisco: Jossey Bass.

Fonteyn, M & Cahill, M (1998). The use of clinical logs to improve nursing students' metacognition: A pilot study. J Adv Nurs 28(1), 149-154.

Gonda, BJ (1990). Nursing student perceptions of learning environments in associate and baccalaureate postconferences. Unpublished doctoral dissertation. New York: Columbia University Teachers College.

Hays, BJ (1994). The new paradigm: Concepts and application in community health nursing. Public Health Nurs 11(3), 150-154.

Kielinen, CE (1997). Journaling; An opportunity for reflection. ABNFJ 8, 8-10.

Letizia, M, & Jennrich, J (1998). Development and testing of the clinical postconference learning environment survey. J Adv Nurs 14(4), 206-213.

Mayo, K (1996). Social responsibility in nursing education. J Holist Nurs 14(1), 24-43.

Murray, JP (1989). Making the connection. Teacher-student interactions and learning experiences. In EO Bevis & J Watson (Eds). Toward a caring curriculum: A new pedagogy for nursing (pp 189-215). New York: National League for Nursing.

Oermann, MH, & Gaberson, KB (1998). Evaluation and testing in nursing education. New York: Springer.

Pierson, W (1998). Reflections and nursing education. J Adv Nurs 27(1), 165-170.

Redmond, GR, & Sorrell, JM (1996). Creating a caring learning environment. Nurs Forum 31(4), 21-28.

Sellappah, S, et al. (1998). The use of questioning strategies by clinical teachers. J Adv Nurs 28(1), 142-148.

Sorrell, JM, et al. (1997). Use of writing portfolios for interdisciplinary assessment of critical thinking outcomes of nursing students. Nurs Forum 32(4), 12-24.

Tanner, CA (1990). Reflections on the curriculum revolution. J Nurs Educ 29, 295-299.

CHAPTER 5

Preparing Students for Home Visits

Christine T. Blasser

Dedicated to my husband Edward F. Blasser, MD, RADM (Ret. USPHS)
December 13, 1927–January 26, 1999
A True Friend Who Cheered Me On

Learning Objectives

1) Discuss the complexities of home visits.
2) Identify key components of faculty preparation and organization.
3) Anticipate student anxieties in making an initial home visit.
4) Consider the impact of preparing students for home visits on the future of community-based nursing.
5) Describe settings where home visits may occur.
6) Describe cultural and personal issues that confront students in community-based nursing.
7) Identify key components of preparing students for home visits.

Out of the corner of my eye I saw the cat carefully lay a gray mole outside the sliding glass door. It was clearly intended as a gift for the drunken owner of the cat, who was in the process of being admitted to a home-health agency. The woman being admitted had a half-gallon of sherry carelessly hidden under a sofa cushion where she had been sitting. She reeked of alcohol. We sat at the kitchen table going through the admission process.

The woman was ataxic and had obviously done some severe neurological damage to her central nervous system through her alcoholism. She was tough looking and was no beginner to drinking. Her speech was slurred. Perhaps she had managed to avoid Adult Protection Services, but most likely had come to their attention at some point—this woman was obviously an advanced alcoholic and had long ago burned all her bridges with family support. I was the mental health nurse who was going out to assess the situation after her doctor had called our office requesting our services. She had fallen and we were to "check her over" for injuries, which was a ruse to get us in the door to see what was really going on. She was not "homebound"—she could drive her car to the closest place to buy her sherry. Luckily she was not a Medicare client and being homebound was not an issue, but the driving in this condition sure was.

I love all animals. I walked over to the sliding glass door and looked down. The little mole lay perfectly still while the cat watched from her proud recline a few feet away. I made a decision. I opened the sliding glass door to quickly grab the mole with a paper towel and remove it to the woods behind the house. The moment I opened the door, it came to life and ran in the house and the real chase began. My blood pressure soared and the client howled with laughter. At this point, I wondered who had better judgment—the intoxicated client or me.

Now I was in deep trouble. I ethically could not let vermin run through the house of a vulnerable person now my client, especially since I was responsible for letting the mole in. On the other hand, how could I explain a "mole bite" to my supervisor? Do moles even bite? I knew I had to now catch the darn thing myself.

I was supposed to complete an admission in a maximum of 1-½ hours. That may sound like a lot of time, but it isn't when you run into psychosocial disasters and intoxicated, sick clients. I began a wild chase after the mole. I envisioned myself as an enlarged Alice in Wonderland frantically chasing after the mole. The poor thing ran under the sideboard in the dining room, but I somehow chased it into the kitchen. It ran behind the refrigerator. I was so frightened I could have lifted the refrigerator. I grabbed a broom and grocery bag. I laid the bag in front of the space beside the refrigerator and wiggled the broom on top of the space. The mole ran in the bag and I grabbed the bag. Somehow I had caught a mole with my ingenuity and bare hands.

The title of this chapter is almost an oxymoron. It can be done, yet it can't be done. There are just too many variables in each home, let alone each client. There are contradictions, and rules sometimes don't apply. In a way, faculty are preparing students not to be prepared, but in an organized manner. Preparing nursing students for home visits requires the faculty to teach the student basic assessment skills and some technological skills, and to activate the student's experiential knowledge and critical thinking. It can be intensely autonomous work. It is the duty of the instructor to help unleash thinking from lockstep formulas used in institutional nursing to thinking that uses creativity and improvisation. Home visits will be unique and rarely repeated encounters in an environment over which the nurse has little control. Reflective practice and continuous learning are the keys to success. Yet all of this is not random and there has to be a "plan B" at all times. Sometimes you need a "plan C."

With that said, preparing students for home visits presents a great challenge to faculty in that there is no one best way to do so. No two home visits are alike, but there are basic threads that run through them. Although there may be a variety of approaches to preparing students for home visits, the underlying concepts of faculty enthusiasm, preparation, and organization remain the keys to success. Critical thinking and creativity do not cancel out organization and preparation. Organization on the instructor's part is essential because most nursing students feel extremely overwhelmed by even the thought of the initial home visit. Remember that you will be modeling the social and behavioral roles you want the students to master and that your enthusiasm and persistence will be rewarded with successful home visits.

FACULTY PREPARATION AND ORGANIZATION

Developing a Preplan

To prepare students for home visits in a variety of settings, you will have to first prepare and organize yourself. If you have not had much experience with home visits or need to refresh your experience, you may have to arrange to work with a nurse mentor who does home visits, such as a home-health nurse, a parish nurse, or a community health nurse. School health nurses are very good resources. Contact agencies early so arrangements can be made.

Once you feel comfortable making home visits in the community in which you will be working, you will be able to convey your confidence to the nursing students. The biggest obstacle you will face is the student's initial fear of failure and self-doubts about being capable of making a home visit. This is not an unusual feeling. Neal (1998) describes novice home-health nurses or "Stage I"

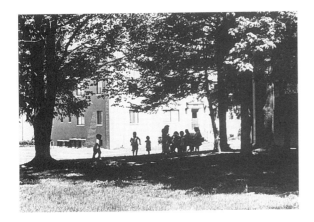

> **Box 5-1** Learning Exercise for Faculty Use
>
> **Developing a Newsletter**
>
> Using a newsletter format, design a newsletter to include information you would want to impart to staff at a community site. Develop a newsletter for the students. Name your publication.

nurses as "overwhelmed and frightened" by the prospect of having to perform competently in the home. Davis (1993) found that nursing students faced very similar feelings and preferred highly structured home visit preparation, and preferred highly detailed and organized learning conditions and close, personal contact with the instructor. Your early investment of time in setting up and preparing for the clinical experience is more likely to achieve increased student satisfaction and achievement.

As early as possible you should know the clinical sites you will be using so you can contact someone at the agency to start your process of preparation. Early faculty contact with the community setting is essential to developing a preplan and allows ample time to begin to learn about the community setting where you will be making home visits. It is imperative that you know the structure and mission of the agency, along with a key contact, so you can establish ongoing communications. Also, find out the agency's expectations of faculty and nursing students as early as possible to avoid unrealistic expectations.

Communication, Communication, Communication

Sometimes another instructor knows the clinical site and can help you get started by sharing his or her information and notes from a previous clinical. Communication is extremely important in the early stages of preparation to establish trust and learn the culture of the organization's staff, although it is wise to start at the site with a fresh, unbiased perspective. You will need to be consistent in your communication to the staff and agency, and ask for feedback to ensure that the goals and objectives of the course are achieved.

If you are developing a site for home visits, you need to be organized and thorough, keeping complete notes as you go along. Gather all information you can about the agency and community you will be assigned to. Keeping the information in a notebook or on a floppy disc will help you organize names and resources. It is important for you to not procrastinate.

Take notes, and record names, phone numbers, e-mail addresses, and fax numbers for each key person you meet. Electronic mail and faxes are excellent ways to communicate, can save a lot of time, and ensure clear, concise communication. Ask if the agency has a Website, and check it out. You will need to pass on much of this information to the students, which can be done in newsletters to keep your communication to them clear and concise.

The staff at the clinical site is often instrumental in finding appropriate home visits for nursing students. For all of my clinical classes I use a newsletter to back up my communication with students, staff, preceptors, and mentors (Box 5–1). My newsletter is called "Bits and Pieces" or BAP. The newsletter includes a variety of learning options and is a good way to reinforce communication. I usually write each student a detailed BAP at the beginning of the clinical with all the phone, e-mail, and fax numbers along with a contingency plan in case I am unavailable and no one is able to cover my class. Then I write newsletters, as needed, for the students because large units of information arise that need reinforcement. Subsequently, I prepare a detailed BAP with a description of the student's mission, goals, and objectives for the staff. Often there is much confusion about the role of the nursing student in the community, especially in making home visits, and this helps to clear up the confusion. Thereafter, I write a weekly BAP for the staff with updates and information about how the clinical is progressing and how the staff can support the students. For the staff, I always write these for the first time I meet with them and then usually write one once a week for each concerned person the student is working with, such as teachers, nurses, principals, and social workers. Typical BAPs that I sent out to teachers in an elementary school the 1st and 2nd weeks of the clinical follow (Tables 5–1 and 5–2).

When you are working in interdisciplinary settings, assume that very often little is known about nursing education. If this is not addressed early, the confusion will be compounded and communication may break down. This can be a setback. Again, at all times, keep your lines of communication clear, honest, and open.

Table 5-1

Bits and Pieces

From George Mason University Instructor Chris T. Blasser, RN, MSN

Nursing 341 Nursing as a Health Service I

Spring Semester

Dear Teachers,

This is the weekly newsletter I usually get out to all the students, mentors, or teachers in clinical areas. Yes, your school is a "clinical area." It is a clinical area for our students because there are many community health issues in schools; in fact, another name for this course is "community health" course. Nurses usually get experience in community and public health, especially in these times when we are focusing on health promotion and disease prevention. Schools like yours are ideal sites for student nurses.

The student assigned to you is a junior student. Let me back up a little and tell you how the nursing program at GMU progresses. The first 2 years of the BSN program encompass liberal arts courses; the junior and senior years are devoted to nursing courses. The students have taken basic nursing courses and will be or are now taking pharmacology and pathophysiology along with clinical and laboratory classes. It is a difficult time, because the coursework is demanding.

The students always feel ill at ease at first in clinical experiences—this anxiety seems to be very prevalent in nursing students because they learn early about the responsibility they carry. The student nurses at Elementary School are no different—they are wondering what will they have to do and how will they accomplish it. I realize some of you have never experienced a nursing student in the classroom. The students are concerned about how they will teach like you do and what they are supposed to do.

As a starting point, the first thing they must do is observe how you teach. They are to observe your techniques (that are appropriate for the grade you teach), and then use these skills along with their health knowledge and start teaching health-related issues to the class. They should be collaborating with you about the required health issues that need to be taught to your grade. For instance, in certain grades hygiene and dental care may need to be taught. This is what the student needs to be doing. They can also teach health-related skills that you feel should be taught. They will learn how to do "head checks" for lice and other types of screening that occurs in the schools in which they are involved. They need to be creative and "kid watch" so they can point out concerns to you. They can do something like this on each day they are in your room. They have access to the library and materials room to get information and create interesting lessons. They will need to make home visits as soon as they can be organized.

The students should be giving you a calendar of when they are in the classroom and when they are in other areas. I will be around to meet you very soon. Please let me know of any questions or ideas you have.

Communication letters can also be used to relay information to the community. This is what we distributed to the parents of elementary school children concerning an asthma project we were developing (Table 5–3). Make sure you clear all communications you send out into the community with the agency where you are based. When the community includes residents whose first language is not English, remember to prepare translated versions in the appropriate language.

Details

Ask the agency contact person if you can attend a new employee orientation, or part of one if time is a constraint, or visit the site to do a "needs assessment" (basically, find out what you need to know). Many agencies have a nurse assigned to orientation, and, if not, there may be a staff educator who can give you the information you will need initially. Being interested and enthusiastic will go a long way toward establishing good communication and developing trust. Preplan activities include assessing the agency's

- orientation program to the facility and agency for both faculty and students
- expectations for faculty and nursing students
- office policies and practices
- focus for home visits
- staff culture

Table 5-2

Bits and Pieces #2

From George Mason University Instructor Chris T. Blasser, RN, MSN

Nursing 341 Nursing as a Health Service I

Dear Teachers,

I think I have met most of you; if not, I will be around to meet you today, and at the latest on Thursday. All of the students now feel much more comfortable being in a classroom—it is an entirely new experience for them. They will still be observing your techniques of teaching, but they can start doing health-related projects in the classroom this week.

There are several assignments the student nurses have to do. They have to write journals daily, to describe for me how they are using certain concepts (health assessment, etc.), therapeutic communication, epidemiology, communication, and collaboration, along with other professional concepts. They have to write three process reports (this is a "he said, I said, I felt" evaluation-type report). They have one graded health project using nursing and health concepts along with a required paper. Attendance is mandatory unless they have a medical excuse or very good other excuse. Their clinical behavior is assessed. I will be speaking to you about this. Please let me know of any problems in this area. They are required to do a home assessment.

An exciting project that we will be doing is the Asthma Project. This is a project that has several parts, including one for the students at Elementary School. A post graduate student and I will be formulating a plan this week to start on this. What we will be doing is case-finding students who have asthma and have no health-care provider, and thus rely on episodic care in the emergency rooms. This project can be viewed as a pilot, although it is not a research project at all. We will probably have to limit the size of the project to either the student's home classrooms (your room) if there are enough students who fit our criteria, or to all kindergarten and or first grade. After we have identified the cases, the students will then start doing home visits to assess the homes and environment and to begin teaching to students, families, and small groups. We hope ultimately to help get the children connected with medical providers and promote self-care abilities to the children and families in the management of asthma. This project should not be a problem because we are in the school until May. Hopefully, the public health department will pick up and continue the project if this works out.

Thank you very much for taking a student in your classroom. Student nurses seek this clinical experience, and we always have more requests to come than we can take. Your superb teaching and advocacy for the students at your elementary school is well respected at GMU.

Table 5-3

Communication Letter

George Mason University

Nursing 341 Section 205

March 3, 1999

Dear 1st Grade Parents at Elementary School,

There are George Mason University student nurses at your child's elementary school for the spring semester. They are learning to be nurses and need to visit some of the students' homes to understand about health issues. We are especially interested in families with children who have asthma.

Asthma is a disease that causes breathing problems like wheezing and shortness of breath. Asthma may hinder children from participating in some activities. Asthma should be treated by a medical professional on a regular basis, and there are certain medications that may be used to prevent lifelong problems.

If your child has asthma and we know about this, one of the George Mason University student nurses may be contacting you about coming out to your home to ask you some questions and tell you about asthma. If you agree, the student will come at a time convenient to you. Your cooperation may help us better understand and treat asthma.

If your child has asthma and the teacher or school nurse is not aware of this, please let them know. We may be contacting you next week about a home visit.

Thank you for your cooperation.

Sincerely,

- perspective on how the students should be prepared by the faculty
- housekeeping issues; for instance, closings, inclement weather plans, parking, rooms where you can meet with students, and basic security expectations and issues.

The students always notice my organization and preparation in clinical settings, and this seems to alleviate some of their initial anxiety, for they seem to think, "at least someone knows what he or she is doing." The vast majority of my students want structure at first, which I initially deliver by my personal preparation and good organization of the information I am going to teach.

Knowing the Community

Faculty must take into consideration many variables that will affect the preparation of students. These include the type of agency, socioeconomic factors of the area, experiential knowledge and learning needs of the students, focus of care and purpose of the visits, and the demographics of the recipients of care.

One of the easiest ways to get a good perspective of the demographics is by visiting a Website. Often local governments and schools have well-developed Websites where you can get a good overview of the area and its demographics. Local government, business, and charitable agencies often have offices that serve the community where you can get information on the services that are available free or for minimal cost to qualifying persons. Many communities offer a guide to services. A very good source of information in any community is through social workers and newsletters that are directed at populations you will be working with, for instance, school newsletters or senior-citizen newsletters.

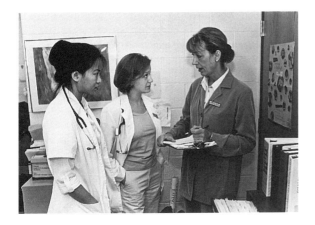

THE LEARNER'S PERSPECTIVE: YOURS AND THE STUDENTS'

As a faculty member, the first item on your agenda is to assess the student's learning needs and experiential knowledge about home visits. Keep in mind that preparing nursing students for home visits is not like following a recipe, but more like creating a recipe using interesting ingredients and going about it in both a logical and creative way. There is no place other than home visits that will call upon an integration of your experiential knowledge, organizational skills, and wisdom to teach, along with the same from the student.

If you have not had recent home visit experience yourself or prepared students for home visits before, you may want to review a more comprehensive text on homehealth visits. You will quickly realize that home visits are a unique area of practice that may produce an overwhelming feeling of being alone, somewhat like being a little dinghy on the ocean with no rudder. Analyzing home visits into stages is one convenient method to allay some of these feelings, because it allows for careful preparation. Although all the stages are important, the previsit stage is very important because it helps to clarify the unknowns.

Stages of a Home Visit

The following section outlines three stages of home visits, and each stage builds on the preceding one. They are the previsit stage, the visit stage, and the postvisit stage. Whenever possible, the faculty member should plan on accompanying the student on the initial visit to a home. At first this may seem like an impossible feat, but when home visits are arranged early in the semester and scheduled on a regular basis to allow sufficient time for each visit, this can be done. Faculty can talk students through the stages of a home visit before it occurs; doing this in the preconference will help the other students think through the process. The student may be assigned with another student for the second visit. If a journal is being used, the three stages of the second visit can be described there for faculty review.

Keep in mind that these stages reflect the nursing process and help students develop a clear nursing perspective and develop nursing diagnoses. Requiring students to either discuss the visit in detail or prepare written plans often helps students overcome any initial fear of the visit. To be effective, home visits demand organization and good time management, as well as physical and mental preparation. A nursing student's home visit should include the following activities in each stage:

Previsit Stage

- State goals and objectives for the home visit.
- Review available records of client.
- Anticipate the plan of care to be given.
- Gather educational materials if available or develop appropriate materials.
- Make arrangements for the home visit, including time and directions to the home.
- Plan the route to the home using a map.
- Coordinate the visit with a translator if necessary.
- Prepare equipment if necessary.
- Review assessment forms.
- Identify potential nursing diagnoses.
- Review safety and environmental concerns.
- Communicate visit time and logistics to faculty (or responsible person at agency) in writing and orally.

Visit Stage

- Initiate social phase.
- Begin assessment phase.
- Validate potential nursing diagnoses.

- Start implementation phase.
- Coordinate planning phase (for next visit) and arrange time.
- Summarize outcomes of the visit and future plans for the client(s).
- Evaluate what the client learned or the outcomes of the visit.

Postvisit Stage

- Return any equipment or educational materials.
- Review nursing diagnoses.
- Document all activities.
- Communicate information to appropriate staff.
- Coordinate referrals if appropriate.
- Formulate evaluation of nursing student (self-evaluation and faculty evaluation)

The Guide at the Side

Most students rely on and expect the faculty to model appropriate clinical behavior. Initially there may be a great deal of dependence on the faculty for direction, especially in making home visits. This seems to parallel Neal's (1998) three-stage process towards autonomy in home health. It is helpful for the faculty to frame the process as it is noted to all students before they make an initial home visit. These stages are

- **Dependence:** In this stage all of the nurses feel overwhelmed and frightened about the logistics and their clinical skills to make a home visit.
- **Moderate dependence:** In this stage there is movement towards autonomy, and the anxiety level is reduced. The nurse continues to ask questions, but this has decreased.
- **Autonomy:** The nurse becomes comfortable with his or her skills and time management. The nurse now consults with others when issues and questions arise.

Although this is a simplified version of the process, it closely parallels how nursing students progress toward autonomy. Home visits require autonomy and good critical-thinking skills. Unlike institutional nursing where "someone is always at your elbow," in the home visit, someone is a phone call away. In the community, nurses are challenged to use peers in more creative and resourceful ways.

Home visits require independent decision making and autonomous actions, heavily relying on the use of critical-thinking skills. Home visits offer an excellent opportunity for nursing students to learn on their own and develop independence and critical-thinking skills. The following shows how Eric felt about his first home visit:

As a nursing student, my first experience doing a home-health visit was terrifying.... What would I say? How would I act? How would I begin to physically examine my client? What if he doesn't like me? These were just a few of the thoughts racing through my mind as I walked up the driveway and into my client's home.

Being a "guide at the side" cannot take away the self-doubts and fears the student will undoubtedly experience at least on the first home visit. The lesson learned will be that home visits can be fun, interesting, and eye-openers to the health needs of the community. Here is another observation from a home visit:

I learned a lot about myself from my home visit. When I originally met the family in the office, I felt they were noncompliant and did not care about seeking help. The daughter is 4 and has a diagnosis of asthma.

When I went to their home, I realized the 4-year-old and her mother were very scared and frightened. The mom is from another country and has no money, no husband, and no job. She is scared and too afraid to ask for help. I learned never to prejudge a situation.

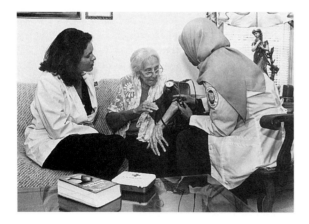

> **Box 5-2** Learning Exercise for Faculty Use
>
> ### Family Scenario
>
> Design a critical-thinking exercise with a family scenario including the variables of poverty and noncompliance. Include the concept of assumptions in thinking and how one can become more aware of assumptions.

IMPLICATIONS FOR HEALTH-CARE CHANGE

The purpose of home visits is varied but revolves around assessment, health promotion, disease prevention, and the treatment of acutely and chronically ill clients. Home visits provide an excellent experience for students to participate in "finishing the story" or continuing the inpatient care provided by other nurses (Neal 1998). Greater emphasis in health care in the future will be health promotion and illness prevention, including client education—in other words, being proactive versus reactive about health issues. Nurses of the future will be expected to increase the focus on health education and to provide and interpret information to clients and families (Oermann 1994). Community-based care will be used as an alternative to longer hospital stays, requiring the nurse to provide more acute care in the home. As is commonly heard in the hospitals, clients are being discharged "sicker and quicker" after having received "drive-through surgery."

After many years of focusing nursing students to be prepared for high-tech facilities (institutions such as hospitals), educators are now increasing their efforts to prepare students for community-based nursing. This trend has been the result of changes in health-care payment and has greatly affected the recipients of care—the individual, family, and community, as well as providers of care—nurses and other health-care providers. Many nursing school curricula are in transition from an acute-care institutional focus to a community-based focus. In the future, more nurses will be practicing in the community because of the changes in health-care delivery—decreased average patient stays in hospitals, shifting of funds to home care, and increased emphasis on health promotion and illness prevention. An effective program that provides students with positive opportunities and challenging experiences in home visits might lead to an increased interest in employment in the rapidly expanding field of community-based nursing (Happell 1998).

Nursing student participation in settings that offer home visits can be used to widen the scope of services and, through the eyes of a novice, provide a unique perspective to help develop proactive versus reactive strategies to improve health-care delivery in the home (Happell 1998). Although students sometimes view community-based nursing as boring and less sophisticated than hospital nursing, clear objectives can help students have clear expectations of what is to be accomplished in a home visit. Students in large home-health agencies will have the opportunity to observe that many health-care professionals are now providing care in the home (including physicians), and the level of skills needed are comparable to those needed in intensive care units. As often heard in home-health settings "those (patients) who used to be dead are in ICU and those who used to be in ICU are at home."

Another perspective to instill in students is the opportunity to make a difference in health care through teaching small groups. Overall, national health education campaigns have not been successful. It is conceivable that consistently providing health education to smaller groups with more pertinent and timely information can be more effective. Nurses possess the knowledge and skills needed for providing health education to groups.

One aspect of community-based nursing, home-health care, can be promoted through the development of challenging and productive home visit experiences, whether for assessment or for direct nursing care. A sincere effort on behalf of the educator to concentrate on the positive aspects of home visits, maintaining a sense of humor, adventure, and enthusiasm helps too. A gentle reminder to the students about the conceptual and historical underpinnings of nursing in relation to the delivery of care in the home and community may be in order.

There is definitely a learning curve in making home visits, both for nurses with institutional experience, as well as for nursing students. The faculty needs to stress perseverance and fortitude. Although making a career in home-health care may not be for many nurses, we can influence the attitude of nurses willing to try this area of nursing practice when a positive experience as an undergraduate is provided.

WHERE HOME VISITS OCCUR

First of all, we must keep in mind that home can be defined in a variety of settings. Home can be a family's place of residence, a house, the social environment formed by the family, a congenial environment, a place of origin, or an establishment providing residence and special care for disabled persons. Homeless persons may reside in a shelter or in a park, under a bridge, or elsewhere in temporary settings, which is then their home. Others may live in transient places such as a migrant worker camp or in an apartment occupied by several immigrant families. A home to many is not what you or I may envision, but symbolically it has the universal idea of a safe haven where we are rooted in our world. This is what one of my students said about a home visit:

> *The home visit I went on definitely differed from what I had expected. Most of the time we hear of home visits being done at poor, run-down homes. We are told as students to be prepared for the worst conditions and unsanitary environments. The populations mainly assessed in our clinical have been of a lower socioeconomic status. So, it was much to my surprise when I got to the home at which I was doing my home visit—it was practically a mansion.*
>
> *I was assigned to be the case manager of this particular VIP client because "he has dementia." I was the mental health nurse for the home-health agency, and this quickly aroused my suspicion. The client was a VIP living outside Washington, DC. Intuitively I felt there must be something wrong here because there was no diagnosis of dementia on the client's chart. In fact, when I first met him, his grace and intelligence struck me. I silently assessed his mental status, and all seemed normal. I quickly realized the other nurses were afraid of him because of his reputation and prestigious career.*

> *There were rules when I entered the home. I would knock and be let in by the housekeeper who would show me to the library. I would sit in one of a pair of chairs beside each other. I would not face the client. This was almost the inner sanctum of the client, and you had to play by his rules, which were obviously "détente." I played along and had a great relationship with the client.—Author*

Nurses making home visits are guests in the client's home. Just as if we were visiting a friend, we must remember to ask permission before we do something and be courteous and considerate to the homeowner or dweller. Anyone who has a "take charge" attitude will quickly get into a no-win situation. At any time the client has the right to refuse a home visit. The client may listen attentively to directions coming from a "talking head" but may decide not to follow up because of the attitude conveyed by the nurse and the way the information was presented.

Cultural Diversity in the Home

In most parts of the country there have been influxes of people from all over the world, but this is especially noticeable in urban areas. Cultural differences will be evident in many situations, and we as nurses and other health-care workers need to be respectful of them. How we communicate both verbally and nonverbally develops the basis of a relationship that either is a success or a failure. For instance, your nonverbal and verbal reaction to a strange or disagreeable odor on first entering a house may affect your relationship with the client. Be especially aware of facial expressions, both yours and the client's. Often clients from cultures different from the nurse will not verbally communicate because it is too assertive a method for them, but much communication will be conveyed through facial expressions and metacommunication.

Personal Boundaries

An important issue that has to be addressed in the home relates to professional boundaries. Seasoned home-health nurses have issues with this, and issues often arise with nursing students. As Coffman (1997, p 2) expressed, there is a "double-edged effect of the support rendered by home nurses and the invasion of family privacy" in the home. In hospitals and institutions it is much easier for the nurse to set up clear boundaries; after all, she or he is in charge of the environment, and clients are separated from the home. In the hospital, the focus is on the biomedical aspects of the disease, whereas, in the home, the focus is often psychosocial (Coffman 1997). Neal (1998, p 273) makes some observations about nurses in the home "walking a fine line." The following dichotomies illustrate the "fine lines" between

- being professional and forming a client friendship
- being a guest and an intruder
- being accustomed to directing the client (autonomy) and respecting that the client is in control
- relinquishing control (autonomy) to the client and being responsible for outcomes
- being supportive of the client and knowing when to disengage from the client
- directing client care and following physician recommendations
- being involved in the client's life and being respectful of the client's privacy.

A home visit can be very stressful to the client and family involved. The nurse may be seen as upsetting the dynamics of the home and may actually arouse defense mechanisms by the client and family that blur the lines of professional behavior. The nurse needs to pay attention to client behaviors and his or her boundaries, and then discuss them with nursing students. This will be the mortar that helps model essential professional behaviors in the home.

Clear agency and professional expectations will aid both the nursing student and client with boundary issues. The student who has clear objectives for a home visit should be better able to communicate to the client the purpose of the visit and what may and may not be accomplished.

PREPARING STUDENTS FOR HOME VISITS

A well-prepared faculty member enhances student-faculty trust. Even an experienced faculty member does not know everything there is to know about home visits. Therefore, successful home visits require an open mind and "LOJ"—learning on the job for both you and the student, and most of all, expecting the unexpected.

 I heard the peculiar sound of roosters crowing as I walked into the ranch-style house in the suburbs. I looked around for the cuckoo clock. It happened again. This time I smelled chickens, and there was no cuckoo clock. The homeowner had two pet chickens in cages on the enclosed porch that she had raised from chicks that her grandson had brought home from school. They crowed every time a new person came to the house.—Author

Not every student will be lucky enough to witness the variety of pets I have seen in homes (squirrels, pit bulls, rabbits, and lizards, just to name a few). Home visits really can be very interesting and exciting—yet, one has to be prepared for almost anything. Again the faculty's enthusiasm, preparation, and organization can help to mitigate any fears students may have about home visits.

Because home visits usually take place during the community-based clinical, there should be time to assess individual student learning needs and preferences, and then to devise teaching strategies to ensure learning takes place. The most important aspect of preparing students for home visits is developing a bond with each student. Bonding leads to trust, which in turn leads to student confidence in what you do and say. You will be a role model for at least the first home visit for each student. Although some students may have had some prior experience making home visits and will be more comfortable than others, some will need more modeling than others. Once students observe your techniques, they usually are able to utilize the innate skills they most likely already possess to conduct a home visit. They will just need practice.

Laboratory Practice for Home Visits

As you get to know your students, you need to assess their experiential knowledge about home visits and the community. Some of the students will have had first-hand experience, and some will have fixed ideas or no preconceived ideas about making home visits. Structured learning situations can be very helpful in getting students over the initial fear of home visits. If a supply or nursing bag will be carried on the visit, then bag techniques will need to be taught. Determine whether the agencies involved will orient you and the students to their specific practices, but remind nursing students about fundamental nursing techniques of washing the hands first, utilizing standard or universal precautions, and going from clean to dirty. At the junior level in community-based nursing programs, the nursing students are usually focused on health promotion, disease prevention, and family assessments. The home visit plans are framed in the steps of the nursing process and the development of nursing diagnoses. There is also emphasis on coordination of care across disciplines. The students need to be aware of resources in the community, and must collaborate with providers in the community to access services available.

At George Mason University (GMU), there is a "blitz" to prepare students for the community clinical. The instructors have the opportunity to meet with their students on two days that are designed to orient students to the various agencies and community resources and safety issues. Time is allowed for individual instructors to meet with their students. This is a good time to discuss home visits and how the goals and objectives of the course can be met through home visits. The home visit assessment form used in community-based nursing programs usually assesses several factors in the home, including health assessment, functional assessment, psychosocial and financial resource assessment, environmental assessment, and cultural assessment. The family is asked to define the health issue(s), and then to work with the nursing student to develop solutions for identified health concerns. At all times the goal of the nurse in home visits is to teach and promote self-care. The public health agencies are usually involved, and the students will often have a separate orientation to these agencies, reviewing the role public health nurses have in community-based nursing. This is a good time to review the home visit assessment form you will be using with the students. Usually the first day in the community site is reserved for orientation.

A simulated home visit in a laboratory can be very helpful to students. The lab can be set up with a range of issues that students may be exposed to including safety and environmental factors. The instructor role-plays the client, and the student conducts the family assessment to practice technique. Students can then practice on each other until they feel comfortable with the assessment and documentation. Students need to practice taking notes during the assessment and documenting the assessment as soon as possible after leaving the home. A review of therapeutic communication skills is also very helpful in teaching students assessment expectations.

Usually you will have a preconference and postconference on each clinical day. These may last 30 to 45 minutes, and they provide time to discuss daily learning objectives and concerns that may arise in the clinical area. Short, written assignments serve as one strategy to help students develop critical-thinking skills by using "what if" scenarios and then discussing these in the group. Once students start questioning their responses and assumptions to clinical issues, they begin to approach problems as a challenge to creatively use information they learned in the classroom, integrated with practical knowledge and wisdom.

The postconference is used to discuss students' concerns and perceptions about what they encountered that day. Often, there are emotional issues, because students may observe things in the home that may be unsettling. The postconference needs to be a safe, supportive environment for students to learn how to handle their emotions and develop lifelong strategies. Lastly, there is a time and place for almost everything in life. Humor and the ability to release tension by sharing laughter and to laugh at ourselves is a remedy that can be modeled.

Helping Students Complete a Community Assessment

Prior to practicing in the community and going to homes, students need to conduct a community assessment. This assessment includes a windshield survey of the community, investigating the demographics and socioeconomic factors of the community, exploring the resources available in the community, and assessing the needs of the community. Students should do the community assessment as early as possible to better serve the clients with whom they will be working.

In our community, the county government prints a small handbook with the names and addresses of most local, county, and national government and nonprofit agencies that offer services in the community. Community-based nursing is an exercise in interdisciplinary health care, and students can begin to learn to build bridges with other disciplines that work for the betterment of community health. Students can do site visits to agencies as they assess needs in their clients. My favorite saying to my students is, "shake the plum tree." One of my students responded by collecting over 400 toothbrushes that were donated for a dental-hygiene program in the elementary school where we did a clinical. The information students accrue can be used to coordinate client care and to educate clients about the availability of services in the community and how to access them. A thorough knowledge of the community resources provides the students with essential information to enhance their practice in the community.

Maps of cities and communities are basic tools the students will need to learn how to use. Make sure you assess the student's knowledge of using street maps and plotting where they are going. Students from another culture may need some individualized time to learn about navigating in the community.

UTILIZING THE NURSING PROCESS IN HOME VISITS

The nursing process can be fully utilized to prepare students to make home visits. The framework includes

- Assessing before the home visit is made: collecting information from records and others who participated in care.
- Formulating nursing diagnoses based on differences among actual, risk, possible, and wellness nursing diagnoses.
- Identifying outcomes based on client considerations and problem identification with formulation of measurable and realistic goals.
- Planning a written plan of care with a summary for the client. The plan will direct student activities in providing health promotion and disease prevention in the home visit.
- Implementing the nursing care plan (on the first visit). Usually more than one home visit is necessary to initiate the plan of care.
- Recording the response to the plan of care, reassessment, and evaluation of the response.
- Evaluating the care delivered—judging the success or failure of the plan of care and the attainment of client goals.

The nursing process, an important framework for nursing care planning, encourages nursing students to learn accountability and to use professional nursing standards and critical-thinking skills. As students become more comfortable making home visits and preparing assessments and plans of care using this framework, they can begin to incorporate critical-thinking skills and build on existing thinking skills.

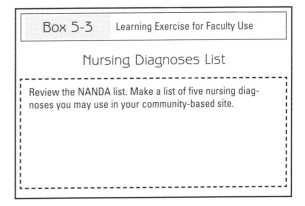

Box 5-3 Learning Exercise for Faculty Use

Nursing Diagnoses List

Review the NANDA list. Make a list of five nursing diagnoses you may use in your community-based site.

Rules and Regulations

Because there are many agencies where you could potentially be assigned, you will have to determine the rules and regulations of that agency and become knowledgeable of the nursing program policies. For instance, for insurance liability reasons, most nursing programs prohibit the faculty from transporting students or clients in their vehicles and students from transporting clients. Many agencies have similar rules.

Another issue is student presence in clinical areas at times other than the regular hours. For example, determine the school policy regarding scheduling home visits on weekends or in the evenings. Are students being allowed to make solo home visits (without you or with another student) at times outside the regular hours? Usually the faculty member has to be present in the agency or available by phone or pager. Both you and the students need to know the practice parameters in the clinical area. Usually school and agency rules and regulations will affect you and the students. You will be prudent to thoroughly understand the legal implications of all rules and regulations. Communicate them to students both orally and in writing. These issues can be included in the BAP format.

Lastly, accidents and incidents do happen. Hopefully nothing will happen, but if something does, be sure to know the policy on incident reporting—both for the agency and the nursing program. If something does happen, the necessary forms need to be completed.

Documentation of a Home Visit

Documentation of a home visit can range from an entry in an agency log to a complete assessment form designed to cover a broad range of health issues. Because community-based nursing practice is most concerned with the individual, family, and small group, a family assessment form is the standard nursing assessment students complete. As early as possible, students should be supplied with the family assessment form you will be using. This will give them the opportunity to review it and practice using it in the classroom. The form can be included in the course syllabus.

Faculty and students must be aware of the importance of confidentially related to home visits. Families may be reluctant to share information with nursing students, and the families need to be informed about the information that will be documented and with whom it will be shared. Remember that at all times families have the right to decline visits. The previsit stage, when the visit is being scheduled, is the appropriate time for you (or the student) to clarify these issues. Be open and honest, but reassure the families that the home visit is a learning experience for nursing students. This usually allays any fears. For instance, if the home visit occurs through a parish nursing program, the information will be shared with the parish nurse. If the agency is a school, then the information can be shared with the public health nurse for that school. At times, social workers or other health professionals will be involved.

The same standards of documentation exist for recording home visit care as institutional care. Students should at all times use professional language and acceptable abbreviations. Documentation needs to be objective, factual, complete, timely, and nonjudgmental—as your mother so often said, "Never put anything in writing what you wouldn't want the world to read." Students need to practice documentation with this in mind.

Safety and Logistics of Home Visits

Safety, and to a lesser degree, logistics, involves becoming aware of your environment. It is never wise to function on autopilot when working in the community, because that's when errors may occur. Multiple bits of sensory and intuitive information will be bombarding you in a strange environment. This is truly where the "men are separated from the boys" in organization and preparation. Mistakes can be dangerous and costly, but they do happen.

It was one of those Northern Virginia ice storms, and it was moving in fast. I parked my "bulldog" (my old Volvo) on a hill outside the home I was visiting. I had just slammed the door shut when my beloved car began rolling backwards down the hill on the ice! Before I had time to think, I jumped in the car and steered it backward down the hill without getting a scratch on it. Providence was shining on me. When I realized what I had just done, I felt faint.—Author

Cars and their maintenance are major concerns in making a home visit. Although students can walk to some home visits, in other cases, they'll need to use car or public transportation. Each student should have transportation available for home visits. Cars need to be reliable and have locks. Accidents are a major concern when making home visits, especially when trying to find an unknown address in inclement weather.

Preparation for inclement weather includes assessing road conditions and taking such circumstances into account when planning a home visit. Safe driving films are excellent ways to prepare students for road safety. Dressing appropriately and safely for the home visit includes wearing comfortable and "sensible" shoes. Walking shoes that perform well outside and inside the home are *de rigueur*. On occasion, the conditions inside the home may be more hazardous than outside the home.

As stated previously, it is advisable for the faculty to accompany the student to each home for the first time. If there are no safety concerns after this, the student can then make a second home visit with another student. As faculty, you are ultimately responsible for the safety of the students. At all times, a responsible person—staff at the agency—needs to know your or the student's itinerary. A form to document the itinerary is an excellent way to keep track of where students are in the community. The form should include planned departure times and expected times of return. Wireless phones are an excellent safety measure.

Some common safety concerns in making home visits include

- Observation of guns and weapons in the home. Many homes have guns, and often agencies have policies about guns or weapons in the home. It is advisable to review these policies. Often the policy is that staff does not enter homes where there is a loaded gun (it must be removed from the home or unloaded). If there is any question or doubt, don't go until the issue is resolved.
- Notice of vermin in the homes. Vermin may include roaches, so if noted, be careful to avoid leaving with them via bags and clothing. Rodents are a constant problem in urban areas, and students need to be aware of this reality to help reduce the shock of an initial encounter. Common sense in avoidance of contact with all vermin is prudent.
- Not knowing where you are going. A common cause of accidents is not knowing where you are going and trying to figure it out while driving. Trying to read a street map while driving should always be avoided. Students need to get directions from the client, locate the address on a street map, and then write out the directions and estimate how long it will take to get there.
- Violence in the home. If you or the student encounters violence of any sort, leave immediately, and call 911 from outside the home. Students need to have enough change to make a phone call if they do not have a wireless phone available. If you do enter a home with unknowns about safety, it is important to keep a clear path between you and the door. Students need to be reminded to be aware of their intuitive feelings and to respond accordingly.

Planning and Organizing the Home Visit

A clinical instructor in nursing has much in common with a parent. No matter how many times you review the necessity of scheduling the home visit, getting directions, mapping your route, gathering material, coordinating an interpreter if necessary, and estimating the travel time, something may be left out. This is part of the learning process, and it is the best way to learn. Try not to rescue the students and allow them to learn from their mistakes when personal safety is not at stake. After the first visit, students will usually realize how important the details and organization of preparation are.

Although I have stressed the importance of organization and preparation, keep in mind that you and the students will need to remain flexible and adapt readily to change. When plan A does not work out, try plan B. Demonstrating flexibility and adaptability to the students will plant seeds that will hopefully develop into lifelong learning. As nurses, all of us need the ability to make changes as new information becomes available in order to incorporate it into our practice.

Making a Home Visit Happen

During a recent community health clinical, the students were procrastinating and finding excuses why they had not scheduled a home visit. Sometimes when I write things out, I "see" what needs to be done. I kept notes for future reference about some of the frustrations that I encountered with the students and logistics of making a home visit.

The students were unable to get going in making arrangements to do home visits. They seem overwhelmed by starting somewhere and are floundering. Most of the group is finding it easy to avoid because they are all in the same boat. No one has made a home visit so far, and it is nearly the end of the first half of the semester. There were some appointments made, but the families all canceled or were not there when we arrived. We are so busy with projects in the agency, I, too am putting the home visits on the back burner.

At last one student made a home visit that she had scheduled. It seemed to break the spell. She was so proud at being the first to make a home visit. Now the other students have become concerned and they seem to realize they have to make a home visit and time is running out in this half of the semester.—Author

When we returned to the community agency after spring break, I had an idea to try to base home visits on a particular health-care issue, childhood asthma. The students knew a lot about asthma because we were working hard to develop an asthma education program in the school. They had a base of knowledge they shared among themselves. They all were assigned to teach the teachers in the school about asthma. They worked in groups of two, and each group was required to demonstrate its project in a practice session. The other students and faculty were to "evaluate" them and give feedback. This helped the students feel more comfortable about their skills in teaching. We discussed such things as learning styles and making effective visual presentations. Now the students felt confident to teach clients. With a solid background in asthma, they could take their skills into the home on home visits. This is what happened in the second half of the semester.

The same problems with the home visits persisted—cancellations and no one at home. I decided to take action by scheduling a few home visits myself, using asthma survey information we had developed to get leads for suitable home visits. After I did this, things took off, and we started to make headway.

Two weeks into the second half of the semester we had made only 5 home visits out of 13 we had scheduled. Most canceled at the last minute. The students and I had called at least 20 homes. There were many reasons home visits could not be made. The biggest obstacle was the language barrier. If Spanish was spoken we were lucky; we had a student fluent in Spanish. Often, when we called to set something up, there was a message on an answering machine in English, in a home where we knew another language was spoken. The child would usually be responsible to translate the messages for the parents, and there was no follow-up on the parent's or caregiver's part. Many parents refused because they worked long hours and could not make time or take time from work. Sometimes we were able to work around their schedules. If there was no calendar in the house or the parents were illiterate, no note was written for the planned visit and they forgot to be there. Sometimes they changed their minds about having strange people in the house (nursing students and instructors) and left to avoid us without canceling the visit. In some cases, teachers or social workers would go with us, and we would just "show up" at the client's home, hoping someone was there and would be receptive to a visit.

The home visits we did get to make were not one-time visits. It took at least one visit just to build rapport and trust. To build rapport and trust, we always try to meet the person "where he or she is." This means we start where they want to, not where we want to. So the first visit is the "icebreaker." If there are health records available for the students to read before the visit, it really helps. Almost all home visits require at least a second visit to get to the health issues. Once we get into a home, they often want us to return. Now the students could return to the home with another student.—Author

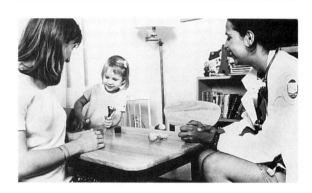

In the homes the students were almost all able to do an assessment on the first visit. The instructor's role in home visits is to guide the student in navigating the scheduling and logistics of the visit, support the student in the assessment phase of the nursing process in the home as needed, assess environmental safety, and do a formative evaluation after the visit.

The student should be prepared to offer educational information and materials.

Most of the families we visit are of lower socioeconomic status. They may have grade-school education, or be totally illiterate. In these situations, immediate survival is usually their chief concern. Our role as nurses is to convince them that we have information that can help them meet immediate needs of survival better and that what we offer is worthwhile. Information needs to be kept simple and interesting. Most importantly, learning readiness must be assessed, as well as their comprehension of the material taught. If they perceive the information as too complex, not immediately useful, or confusing, it will be rejected, no matter how vital the issue is. I needed to provide the student with guidance and planning for educational projects to ensure the use of appropriate learning principles.

Once we get in the home and start talking, we have to be very careful not to overstay our time in the home. It may take a lot of time to get past the social aspects of the visit. Then the student tries to get the family assessment done. If there is a planned teaching program, it may require at least one other visit to get to this.—Author

---

The faculty needs to start planning strategies to find home visits early in the community-based clinical. In some community-based clinicals, finding appropriate home visits are not a problem. Identifying a health promotion or disease prevention issue is a good way for the students to focus and helps them prepare for home visits.

Home visits are complex and unique practice opportunities for nursing students and require coordination of many variables. Nursing students at the junior level may be overwhelmed at the prospect of scheduling, organizing, and conducting a home visit. Key components in home visits include organization, time management, and preparation. Faculty needs to support the student in making the first home visit.

The faculty member needs to prepare and organize for preparing students for home visits by being familiar with both the clinical sites and the community. Faculty and students should conduct a careful community assessment of the needs of the community and identify resources in the community. Good communication among faculty, students, agencies, and communities is essential for the goals and objectives of the clinical course to be met.

Faculty members need to ensure that home visits are challenging and productive. Students may have preformed negative opinions of nursing practice in the community. Home visits are an excellent way to promote the idea of improving the nation's health through delivery of care in a community setting rather than limiting care to institutions.

Preparing nursing students to make home visits requires role modeling of social and professional behaviors by the faculty. There are many cultural, social, environmental, and psychological considerations in making home visits. Written assignments and laboratory experiences can help students prepare for home visits. Safety is an important consideration in making home visits.

Students may be initially overwhelmed by anxiety about making a home visit, which can become an obstacle in achieving a home visit. This is usually quickly dispelled after the first visit. Home visits that are well planned, organized, and interesting can promote interest in future community-based nursing careers.

References

Coffman, S (1997). Home-care nurses as strangers in the family. West J Nurs Res 19(15), 12.

Davis, JH (1993). Evaluation of novice home visitor preparation strategies. J Community Health Nurs 10(4), 249-258.

Happell, B (1998). Student nurses' attitudes toward a career in community health. J Community Health 25(4), 269-279.

Neal, L (Ed). (1998). Rehabilitation nursing in home health setting. Glenview, IL: Association of Rehabilitation Nurses.

Oermann, M (1994). Reforming nursing education for future practice. J Nurs Educ 33(5), 215-219.

CHAPTER 6

Teaching Students in Unstructured Community Settings

Christena Langley

Learning Objectives

1) Define the nature of "unstructured" or "nontraditional" settings.
2) Delineate orientation activities helpful to faculty, agency staff, and students.
3) Outline methods of assessment of student behaviors in community-based settings.
4) Explore evaluation criteria appropriate to community-based settings.

Nurse educators have dealt with ambiguities in clinical settings throughout our history. Traditionally, undergraduate clinical nursing courses combine exposure to actual clients with the application of theories, processes, and skills acquired in previous and concurrent courses. There is often a tension between giving the students enough independence to develop confidence in their critical thinking and safeguarding the clients (and the clinical agencies) from the unintentional errors of the novice. Nursing instructors in public health settings are accustomed to seeing their clinical students for short periods of time (for instance, meeting for a home visit or observing the student teaching a health education class) during the clinical day, but these are often senior-level students who have completed several semesters of closely supervised clinical experiences. As clinical courses include community practice earlier in the curriculum, faculty experience concern about the independence of these more novice students in nontraditional clinical settings. In addition, although these sites provide excellent opportunities for clinical education, the number of students that can be accommodated in one setting is often small, and settings may be geographically dispersed.

Some nursing programs have introduced community-based clinical experiences as part of a traditional clinical rotation so that students are based in an acute-care setting such as a pediatrics unit of a hospital but rotate out for part of the semester to a school, clinic, or recreational setting to gain experience with health promotion activities for children and their families (Palmer 1995). In contrast, the George Mason University (GMU) curriculum includes one clinical course during the second semester of the junior year that is community based and a second clinical course at the senior level that is population focused. The combination of these two courses with the other three clinical courses that take place in acute and long-term care facilities gives our students clinical experiences across the continuum of health care. It also affords the faculty many opportunities for leveling community-based content so that students can move their focus from individuals and families to larger groups and populations within community settings, just as they move from simple to complex cases in acute-care environments. With the increased flexibility of our curriculum, we are able to offer more varied clinical assignments.

During the 6 years that our faculty has been implementing our community-based curriculum, we have learned many lessons. The purpose of this chapter is to share some of those lessons that relate to the challenges of clinical rotations in unstructured settings. These settings offer outstanding learning opportunities for novice students and faculty but demand a great deal of effort from faculty, students, and agency staff members for the experiences to be successful.

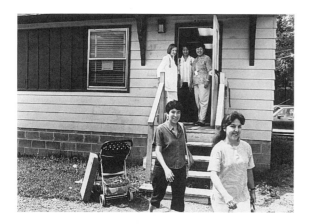

WHAT DO WE MEAN BY "UNSTRUCTURED SETTINGS?"

Once the faculty agreed that we would undertake a junior-level community-based clinical course, our next decision was what clinical sites would be used. We knew that we would need about 10 locations with each being able to accommodate a group of 10 students with an instructor on-site. We are fortunate to be located in a large metropolitan area with many diverse health services. Additionally, our own campus has over 20,000 students, a large faculty and staff, and numerous ongoing community activities crossing the lifespan. We chose to reserve the local public health departments as clinical sites for our senior-level students to achieve their population-focused clinical activities.

We discovered that many of the potential clinical sites in our geographic area are single purpose, or age specific, or offer a discrete set of services that are not broad enough to facilitate student learning at the generalist level. Many are not a part of the traditional "medical" model and lack the traditional nursing management superstructure. They often provide services on a "flex" time schedule rather than the 24 hour/7 day week model of acute-care environments. The services provided are often more "on behalf of" clients (indirect) rather than "hands-on" or technical (direct) services. Many of these agencies rely on allied health professionals and volunteers as an important part of their staff. Services provided are distributive rather than episodic, and staff are often involved in case finding and case management rather than being confined to serving only those people seeking services.

Another challenge revealed to us as we investigated community-based sites was that some of the agencies offer excellent opportunities for nursing activities but cannot accommodate a group of 10 students. Some of these agencies became the "home base" within a network of complementary agencies. Students spend time in each of several (usually two to four) service agencies throughout the semester so that there are no more than six students in an agency at one time.

As we considered a set of clinical agencies (see Chap. 1 for the process of securing clinical sites), we articulated the following assumptions:

- Learning can occur in a variety of traditional and nontraditional health-care environments. Inpatient, outpatient, community-based, and population-focused settings are meeting the needs of culturally and economically diverse clients.
- Staff members in clinical agencies work in partnership with faculty and students to facilitate optimum client outcomes. Interdisciplinary teams of providers enrich the learning experiences of nursing students.
- All of the students will not have the same learning experiences.

Although we knew that in our acute-care clinical rotations our students were not having the same learning experiences, we were comfortable with the commonalties that existed across settings. Certainly, students assigned to an orthopedic unit have different client experiences than those on an oncology unit, but there are themes, such as pain control, that unify the experiences. Similarly, whether students are working in an elementary school with a diverse population of young families, or a psychiatric Club House with chronic mentally ill members, there are also common themes. As Lindemann advised: "...be more flexible and creative in the selection and use of real world clinical settings... (1989 p 66). The goal is to place all of the students in safe environments where they are able to develop clinical judgment and problem-solving skills with opportunities to follow clients across settings.

The common threads of the junior-level community-based course would be: individual and family assessment, health promotion and disease prevention for individuals and families, home and neighborhood assessment, and health teaching for individuals, families, and small groups. Table 6–1 lists several of the categories of sites that offered opportunities to accomplish all of these threads.

In Chapter 1, we described the process of choosing and contracting for community-based clinical sites. Once the contracts are in place, there may be a time lag, however, between the final negotiations and the arrival of the clinical instructor for orientation. As one faculty member observed, this can lead to some unanticipated challenges.

Table 6-1

Examples of Community-based Clinical Sites

Psychiatric rehabilitation centers	Elementary schools
Churches	Senior recreation centers
After-school programs	University campus
Headstart and early intervention programs	Outpatient maternity services
Managed-care providers	Adult day-care centers

When I was arranging my orientation, I learned of the resignations of two of the individuals in leadership positions who had actually made the arrangements for the clinical rotation. No one else on the staff in either of the two settings had been informed that the nursing students were coming. Once arrangements were made and details ironed out, I was in a clinical setting with no previous exposure to BSN students. I was planning on having 10 students rotating through 5 different sites and would not be personally overseeing all of the clinical experiences in each of the sites.

The health-care delivery system appears to be ever-changing, and it is essential to maintain close working relationships among faculty and agency staff to assure positive experiences for students and clients. The clinical instructor needs to be identified well before the beginning of the clinical course to initiate orientation to a new community-based site and to develop contacts with staff members and potential clients.

PLANNING CLINICAL EXPERIENCES

Orientation for Faculty and Agency Staff

Once the clinical site is identified, the assigned clinical instructor becomes responsible for planning the specifics of the experiences. Thorough preliminary planning is essential to a successful semester. Such planning should include several orientation sessions for the faculty member with agency staff before the arrival of the students. In our program, the Clinical Placement Coordinator negotiates the contract for clinical placement with the liaison staff member responsible for student placements in the facility, without spending much, if any, time with staff members who are directly involved in the educational experiences of the students. Therefore, it is extremely important for the instructor to spend time with staff to initiate collaborative relationships that accommodate mutual goal setting and the achievement of shared missions (AACN 1999, Tagliareni & Murray 1995). Here is how one of our faculty members described her preclinical work.

> *There are several challenges when setting up a community-based psychiatric-mental health clinical experience for junior-level undergraduate nursing students. I begin by establishing credibility with staff members, none of whom is a nurse but all of whom welcome our presence in their facilities. Prior to the beginning of the semester, I meet with directors of both centers to explain the course objectives, listen to their expectations of students, share problem solving of potential problems and concerns, and set up the orientation program for the students. At this meeting, I also inquire about possibilities for additional experiences (out-rotations) for the students—for instance, observation in the Clozaril medication clinic, visits to an inpatient psychiatric facility, and so on. I also inquire about any changes in the organization or staffing since the previous clinical rotation.*
>
> *I then schedule a morning in each center, preferably on the same day of the week as our clinical days. At this time, I meet with staff members and spend time in each of the work units where the students will be assigned. This also provides opportunities for me to talk with the members (client or patients). I talk with the liaison staff member identified in each center and begin to forge a relationship. This provides time to clarify clinical objectives and to listen to concerns from previous experiences with students in clinical rotations.*

The instructor will need to become very familiar with the goals, services, and activities of the agency, the roles of its staff members, the demographics of the clients served, and the expectations of the staff for students. Equally important are reimbursement mechanisms, safety issues, and documentation requirements (O'Neil & Pennington 1996). Anticipated issues should be discussed as early as possible so that potential problems can be averted. Often, staff members have had previous experiences with "students" (not always nursing students) and have expectations based on those experiences. The faculty member needs to know this information in advance.

In turn, the staff members need to be oriented to the course objectives, the educational level of the students including what their previous clinical experiences have been, logistical information such as days and hours that students are available, and examples of possible student activities. It is also important for the instructor to share his or her availability. Staff members voice concern that they will be given complete responsibility for the student's learning experience without an instructor available for consultation (Herrman, et al. 1998). During these preliminary planning meetings, the staff members can identify the contact person for the faculty as well as preferred oral and written communication channels. The program for student orientation can be mapped out, including staff who will speak, those who will have students shadow them, and so forth.

Other key issues to be discussed between the instructor and the staff include the following:

- **Student Space.** Despite the cramped quarters of many of the organizations selected for community-based clinical experiences, students need a place where they can gather for conferences with faculty, make phone calls on behalf of clients, work on health education materials, and complete documentation.
- **Student Assignments.** Who will select clients and projects for the students? Ideally the staff, instructor, and students will work together to establish and maintain assignments.
- **Policies and Procedures.** Although nursing students do not need to know all of the details of the organization manual, they need to know their responsibilities especially in the areas of computer access and use, client rights and confidentiality, incident reporting, medication and treatment administration and documentation, and documentation of other activities. The students will be more comfortable if the faculty is knowledgeable of these areas before they arrive for their clinical rotation.
- **Timing Expectations.** Often there are opportunities for students to participate in clinical activities during off-hours that are beyond the hours of the clinical rotation. Staff members and the instructor need to establish the availability of students and faculty member for these types of extended or alternative clinical hours.
- **Orientation for Students.** Unlike acute-care settings where orientation often involves getting an identification badge and parking decal and conducting a scavenger hunt on the assigned unit, community-based clinical sites usually require a lengthier orientation for students. This is in part because of the students' lack of awareness of community-based nursing and the unlimited potential for nursing activities. Community-based sites are often one piece of an interconnected network of agencies with consultation and referral occurring across them. The orientation sessions for students should focus on providing the students with this bigger picture of services as well as the specific rules and regulations of the

assigned organization. The clinical instructor must take an active part in planning the students' orientation so that it is adequate but not overwhelming.

Several different approaches can be useful in making orientation informative but not overwhelming or boring. Students respond very well to interactive activities. A panel discussion by key staff members with opportunities for dialogue is preferable to a series of speakers lecturing to the students. If the panel members have handouts to share with the students, it is helpful if the clinical instructor distributes the handouts in advance so that the students are familiar with them before meeting with the staff. This greatly enriches the dialogue between staff and students during orientation sessions. A written assignment can be used to get at each student's thoughts on such issues as the compatibility of the organization's mission with their own concepts of their social responsibilities in health care.

A mixture of conference activities with scavenger hunts or a windshield survey of the neighborhood also helps to maintain student interest and alleviate fears. Sending the students out in groups of three or four allows them to look at the surrounding neighborhood and identify the location of key services in advance of their solo voyages. One member of each small group acts as the recorder to document their travels and their impressions and reactions.

One of our community-based clinical settings is our university campus. Here is what one clinical instructor recounted about the students' first day.

TOURING

On the first clinical day, I asked the students to do a walking assessment of the campus. The clinical group was divided into four smaller groups and each group explored one quadrant of the campus. That afternoon, we reconvened to discuss their findings and brainstorm about potential clinical activities. They located health-related service offices, health hazards for students and visitors, and accessibility for the handicapped. The group was so creative that we had many more ideas than clinical time!

One of the student-identified goals was gaining experience with the technology of injection administration, so we agreed that each student would participate in Immunization Clinic. We prioritized activities so that all students would be ready to participate in a health fair that was held as part of College Day.

Students collaborated to identify other nursing activities. One was the NURSENERGY health education display table that was moved around on campus from week to week. Weekly themes were chosen to coincide with other university events: "Recognition of Eating Disorders and the Associated Medical Risks" was presented during the university's Body Awareness Week. An outgrowth of the NURSENERGY concept was a weekly health column in the campus newspaper. Members of the clinical group researched and answered health-related questions submitted by university students.

During one of the initial group conference times with students, the clinical instructor gives the group a chance to identify questions about the clinical agency and brainstorm as to which staff member might have the answers. Students can then be assigned to interview these key people and bring information back to the group in an interesting framework. Conference time can also be used effectively to present and review documentation policies as well as forms to be used. The actual use of the forms can be demonstrated through a case study or scenario that requires group or individual work to get at interviewing strategies that would be helpful to ascertain the required information ("overt" versus "covert" information) as well as the decision tree for acting upon information provided. For example, Box 6-1 illustrates how this can be applied with a group of nursing students in Head Start.

Box 6-1   Learning Exercise for Faculty Use

Head Start

A group of students working with Head Start classes need to know the eligibility process. Have the students role play the eligibility interview as part of the intake process. They would first review the eligibility forms. Formulate questions for the interview. Think about ways that they could discover "covert" information. For example, sometimes seemingly innocuous questions about the child's birth and growth will reveal other pertinent information about the family's interaction and needs.

"Shadowing" a staff member for a few hours is a very valuable method of orientation. Each student spends a day or part of a day accompanying a staff member through his or her usual activities. Because students are sometimes reluctant or timid to ask a lot of questions, the clinical instructor can assign a set of questions for the group to ask wherever they go (Table 6–2). The answers can be shared in clinical conference. This is also an effective way to identify different styles of interacting with clients and students exhibited by various staff members. Sharing the information in group conference allows the students to coach each other and benefit from each other's ideas for dealing with staff and clients.

During student orientation, it is also important to schedule some time for group discussion of "professional behavior" issues. Time may be given at intervals throughout the semester to revisit some of these issues as situations arise. Recurring issues center around

- Timeliness—being on time and keeping appointments.
- Appropriate attire—even though they are usually not in white uniforms, students need to dress professionally, limit jewelry, and contain their hair, nails, and makeup.
- Turning off cell phones and beepers.
- Obeying agency regulations about parking, office space, use of telephones, and interrupting staff with questions.
- Eating or drinking in clinical or office areas.
- Safety issues—when surveyed, nursing students report they are fearful of the "unknown" that they may encounter in unstructured or nontraditional community-based clinical sites (Hayes, et al. 1996). They report less fear when they have worked through scenarios and discussed the "what-ifs." Moving from the "controlled environment" of acute care to one where there is little control can be intimidating to students (Carroll, et al. 1999).
- Process of home visiting—an important skill in community-based settings. Students report that accompanying a skilled nurse, social worker, or other health worker on home visits, or making home visits with a student partner or an instructor are extremely valuable to understanding family health issues and developing the skills to work with families. They did not feel that they could get this from simulated role play and reading the literature. (Ford-Gilboe, et al. 1997). It is imperative that the clinical instructor and students have a clear understanding of the agency's policies on safe home visitation and documentation procedures. The clinical instructor must establish

Table 6-2

Examples of Questions for Community Agency Staff

What types of services do you provide?

What is the average number of visits or encounters that you have with clients per day, per week?

How much time do you spend coordinating care?

What are the geographical boundaries of your caseload?

The most common types of health problems in your current caseload are:

The most common case management problems that you encounter are:

Do you have any staff members under your supervision? If so, what are their titles, and how much time per week is spent supervising them?

How much time is allocated for your involvement in in-service opportunities, meetings, or continuing education?

How do you suggest that the students maintain weekly communication with you?

What types of client assignments do you have? What types of activities could you share? How will you refer cases?

clear guidelines for the home visit activities, safe travel procedures, and what to do when a client is not home at the time of the scheduled home visit.
- Confidentiality and ethical issues—smaller community-based organizations often lack the structured record systems of larger health-care providers (Faller, et al. 1995). It is extremely important to develop a clear plan for written documentation for the protection of the vulnerable clients and the staff with whom the students are often working.

Assessment of Students

During the orientation phase, the clinical instructor has many opportunities to begin assessing each of the students in the clinical group. Through their interactions with each other and the staff, the students demonstrate their professional behaviors and some of their strengths as well as limitations in interpersonal communication and group process. The instructor can begin to determine specific clinical assignments that will be beneficial for each student. In addition, the instructor needs to give each student an opportunity to describe his or her personal objectives for this course and perceptions of his or her "best fit" within the activities to be completed during the semester. In our program, with multiple clinical sites to choose from, our faculty discuss with their clinical groups why the students chose to register for a particular section. If there appears to be a mismatch, students are able to trade clinical sites on the first day of clinical when they meet together for orientation to the course.

In addition to discussion, students can use a learning portfolio to demonstrate their past experiences so that the community-based clinical will build upon and augment their previous learning. Adult learners often have multiple years of life and work experience in other settings that can be built on. Through portfolio development and review, the instructor and student can identify other potential problems such as work schedule conflicts that could encroach on clinical hours. It is also important to look at clinical experiences the student may previously have had without an instructor present. How comfortable is each student in performing clinical activities without an instructor being present? In this way, the clinical instructor can begin to prioritize her or his time among the students as well. As they progress through their community-based clinical rotation, students should add examples of their work to their portfolio for reference in future clinical courses.

ONGOING CLINICAL ACTIVITIES

In acute-care settings, clinical students are assigned the nursing care of one to three clients usually as part of one staff nurse's assignment. The student performs the care and communicates with and reports off to the designated staff nurse each day. Many of the activities involve physical care, performance of technologies, and medication administration. In contrast, in community-based settings, many of the activities are done on behalf of clients rather than directly with them, and in collaboration with several staff members, perhaps in different discipline areas. Within our community-based clinical course, students' experiences vary greatly among the different clinical groups. We have identified some common threads to be accomplished regardless of setting: home visiting for assessing individuals and families within their natural environment, health teaching to individuals and families, and health education on a larger scale with groups whose members share a common health interest or problem. Student assignments, therefore, often involve ongoing work with the same individuals or families (health teaching to people coming to the clinic), paired work while making home visits such that one student has primary responsibility with the other acting as observer-recorder, and group assignments (from three members up to the whole group involved) to accomplish a health fair or other type of project.

Time management and prioritization of demands become imperative in a community-based clinical rotation. These skills are often major challenges for students with limited clinical experience that has occurred in acute-care settings with on-the-spot feedback and supervision from an instructor and staff personnel (O'Neil & Pennington 1996). These tasks are also a challenge for the clinical instructor who relies on student encounters throughout the clinical day for both "teaching moments" and "evaluation opportunities."

When they are in the community, students participate in activities when I am not with them. It is difficult to anticipate the "spontaneous moments" of clinical interaction that may occur in an acute-care setting. When the

entire group was on a med-surg unit, I could "pop" into a room and observe what the student was saying and doing. Because of time and distance logistics, I often have to pre-arrange my visits to community-based sites, but I have learned the advantages of varying my routine each week so that I have created opportunities for those "spontaneous moments." The students appreciate my visibility and participation in their clinical activities.

Staff mentors or other role models can greatly facilitate the student's learning if the mentor is open and "able to create an atmosphere where the student can ask questions" (Baillie 1993, p 1048). The mentor does not have to be a nurse, but must demonstrate professional credibility. Social workers and others have much to offer undergraduate students, especially in the areas of collaborative team approaches to health care. The mentor works together with the instructor and student to select clinical experiences and evaluate their outcomes.

Often the clinical sites selected for community-based rotations provide excellent opportunities, but physical settings often are small, and it is burdensome for them to accommodate 10 nursing students on any day. To ease this, the clinical instructor can provide the students with alternative assignments and out-rotations that enhance each student's clinical experience while easing the strain on the home-based clinical agency. These types of assignments are especially useful if the objectives of the course include clients across the lifespan or encompass multiple experiences across diverse groups of clients. We have used networks of related services for subgroups of our clinical groups. Although students in acute-care settings may feel comfortable rotating alone to the operating room from their assigned medical-surgical unit, students in community-based settings prefer to be partnered for an out-rotation (Baillie 1993). They tend to feel isolated if they are the lone nursing student in a community organization, especially if few of the staff members are nurses.

Faculty's Role in Communication

Faculty members need to work closely with students in preparing for clinical activities while providing the actual services, and while accomplishing follow-up activities. One colleague describes this process as a "partnering with students," more of a collaborative-type arrangement than sometimes has previously existed in undergraduate nursing education. Each day, the clinical instructor accompanies students in selected activities and provides continuous feedback. Rather than act as a detached observer, the clinical instructor works together with the student in making the home visit or educating the patients, gradually decreasing his or her role as the student's confidence grows.

Collaborative work with students also changes the dimensions of the clinical conferences. Every week should begin with a short group conference, during which the instructor can assess that each student is on task with prioritizing activities and planning for the week. The instructor will also be able to plan his or her activities based on the discussion in the planning conference. Every week should end with a wrap-up conference to assure that everything is done and documentation is complete. DeLaGarza and Martinez-Rogers (1998) call this the "postclinical debriefing" (p 142) and report its value in allowing students to learn from each other's experiences while assisting each other to plan subsequent actions. In addition, conferences help the students who are slow to catch on to the priorities and time constraints of community-based nursing. Conference time can also be used for other foci, but there needs to be a consistent pattern of accountability exhibited through conference time.

Frequent, brief conferences or e-mail exchanges between the clinical instructor and student greatly facilitate ongoing assessment of each student's performance. The frequent constructive feedback assists the student's growth as a safe and independent nurse. The clinical instructor also needs to schedule frequent interchanges with key agency staff. This may be the principal of the school, the volunteer coordinator in a Senior Center, or the nurse practitioner in a child health clinic—whomever the faculty, staff, and students have designated as the critical communication link. These regular conversations help to identify problems early, brainstorm solutions, and plan ahead based on new opportunities. The staff often uses these scheduled meetings to present ideas or requests for student assignments. One instructor reported that each week in her meeting with the agency supervisor, she received referrals for home visits and requests for health teaching that kept her students busy throughout the semester. The frequency and quality of the requests also communicated to the students that they were valued as an important part of the organization.

STRENGTHENING STUDENT LEARNING IN COMMUNITY-BASED SETTINGS

In acute-care settings, the ultimate goal usually is that the student assumes full responsibility for the total nursing care of assigned clients. In community-based settings, the nursing activities may not be physical care and may involve limited technologies. Rather, the student is moving towards complete responsibility for the planning, implementation, and evaluation of nursing activities done on behalf of the client. This responsibility often involves anticipating activities that cannot be accomplished singlehandedly, and locating and negotiating with appropriate team members for successful collaborative efforts.

Despite the clinical setting, the student remains responsible for obtaining information about the client's current status. It is helpful if students select sample individual, family, and community assessment tools. They will need to begin by thinking, "What do I really know about this nursing care situation?" One group of authors calls this "inquiry-based learning" (Oneha, et al. 1998). Often clients seen in community-based settings do not present with a thick record of histories and physical examinations and lab values for the student to review. Instead, they are seen with brief clinic records, or self-reports in health-teaching classes. Students need to be encouraged to use a combination of "what the client should know" with "what they want to know," while factoring in, "what they already know." The students also need to investigate or review scientific and theoretical content to clarify and further explain clients' situations. Just as in acute care, students in community-based settings must take every opportunity to learn more about pathophysiology, pharmacology, and rationale behind prescribed treatments. Textbooks, periodicals, handouts, pamphlets, and agency manuals can also be helpful.

In acute-care settings, the emphasis is on knowing the pathophysiology and pharmacology in-depth so that the student can perform procedures and administer medications safely; in community-based settings, this information usually provides background information for patient teaching and health education efforts. This background information has to be synthesized with sound principles of health promotion and disease prevention and health education theory to produce teaching materials and sessions that are understood by the clients. The clinical instructor is a vital part of the development of any teaching plan and should preview all handouts, posters, and films or videos to be used for accuracy of content and appropriateness.

Although clinical assignments in acute-care settings are usually accomplished in a fast-paced environment, assignments in community-based agencies require a different organizational style and time management skills. Students in acute-care clinical practicums plan their days around a set of activities that must be accomplished at specific times. In community-based nursing, clinical activities often have to be planned over several weeks and account for daily, weekly, and perhaps monthly activities. Planning ahead and dealing with frequent change can be frustrating for novice students. They may begin with an impression that nothing is time critical and then procrastinate until they are unable to accomplish their assignments by the end of the semester. The instructor needs to be very clear about expectations, which should be communicated both orally and in writing to avoid misunderstandings. Written time sheets can be used to keep a log of activities and hours. This often helps a student identify the need for additional activities or days when time conflicts exist.

The instructor needs to work with the group and each student individually to develop a calendar for the semester (Table 6–3) that shows what needs to be accomplished daily, what activities occur at regular intervals (patient teaching in child health clinic), and what long-term events are pending (the health fair at the elementary school). Time should be allowed for tasks done in preparation for other clinical responsibilities—previewing films to decide which one will be shown to a class or locating educational materials written in a language other than English. Finally, students need to think each week about, "What would be good to do if there is time?" If one activity falls through (a client cancels a home visit, for example), what can I do with that time? Every student needs both a written agenda for every clinical day and a calendar of the whole semester that can be modified as activities change and items are added or deleted.

Table 6-3

Sample Calendar

	PRIOR TO SEMESTER	FIRST 2 WEEKS	ONGOING	FINAL 2 WEEKS
AGENCY STAFF	• Meet with clinical instructor. • Gather handouts for students. • Become familiar with course objectives and student roles. • Outline orientation plan. • Determine space allocation for students. • Think about client assignments.	• Participate in making assignments. • Determine communication routes for students & instructor. • Provide orientation. • Provide opportunities for students to shadow staff members.	• Maintain communication channels. • Assist students to participate in clinical opportunities. • Provide ongoing feedback to instructor and students.	• Identify any outstanding activities that require completion. • Plan and conduct "exit interview/report-off" meeting with students and faculty. • Provide written feedback of the experience. • Confer with instructor and individual students about performance.
STUDENTS	• Obtain map and identify clinical location and best route. • Obtain course syllabus, books, and a calendar. • Update learning portfolio to reflect clinical and life experiences.	• Read course syllabus. • Participate in orientation. • Identify areas of most interest & communicate these to clinical instructor. • Initiate contacts with clients. • Begin developing care/teaching plans.	• Maintain calendar of clinical activities. • Stay on schedule with clinical assignments. • Establish a pattern for clinical hours & maintain journal/log. • Maintain communication with staff mentors.	• Complete all tasks & responsibilities. • Complete all documentation per agency requirements. • Participate in exit meeting. • Complete self-evaluation, & meet with clinical instructor. • Update learning portfolio. • Provide written feedback regarding the course, instructor, clinical site.

Table 6-3   Sample Calendar—cont'd

	PRIOR TO SEMESTER	FIRST 2 WEEKS	ONGOING	FINAL 2 WEEKS
CLINICAL INSTRUCTOR	• Meet with agency staff. • Plan orientation for students with the staff. • Review mission statement and goals of clinical agency. • Spend time (½ day - full day) participating in staff clinical activities. • Outline activities for the students for the first 3 to 4 weeks. • Meet with other faculty teaching sections of the course.	• Review students' learning portfolios. • Initiate goal setting and self-eval plan with students. • Initiate opportunities for partnering with students in clinical activities. • Set up pattern of clinical conferences and individual conferences with students. • Assist students in setting up their calendars. Set up a group calendar.	• Home visit, co-teach, partner with students in clinical activities throughout each clinical day. • Arrange speakers, out-rotations, etc., to enhance students' clinical experiences. • Maintain communication with designated staff members. • Maintain communication with course coordinator, clinical placement coordinator, and other clinical faculty (attend meetings).	• Assure that each student has completed and documented clinical activities. • Return all assignments, graded and with comments. • Provide face-to-face, one-on-one evaluation (as well as written) with each student. • Meet with staff for wrap-up & to plan subsequent clinical rotations. • Meet with course faculty and coordinator to evaluate overall effectiveness of clinical sites, assignments, etc.

The Learning Environment

In traditional clinical settings, students usually are expected to report on and off at the same time each clinical day throughout the semester. In community-based settings where the goal is to bring health care to people in their natural environments, there is a need for more flexibility in students' hours. Opportunities abound following the closing of normal business hours (visits to homeless shelters for screening and teaching, health fairs at public schools in the evenings and on weekends, triaging in urgent care facilities in the evenings); however, such commitments require the instructor and students to adjust their hours to include these activities. (It is also imperative to determine whether the nursing school's liability insurance covers students who engage in clinical activities during "off" hours.)

Clinical instructors need to be supportive and allow students the freedom to test their ideas and abilities. We need to provide affirmation to encourage the students' critical-thinking abilities. We should be assured that students understand terminology by asking questions with several possible satisfactory answers, using open-ended questions, and allowing enough time for the student to think and organize an answer to a question. Most important, we need to provide frequent positive feedback. When it is necessary to deliver constructive criticism, it is important to do so as close in time to the precipitating event as possible, and in a private face-to-face exchange with the individual student.

Clinical Evaluation

Clinical instructors have several other techniques, in addition to direct observation of students engaged in clinical activities, to gather information about their clinical performance in community-based settings. As discussed earlier, individual and group conference time can be extremely useful. A give-and-take discussion of successes and problems encountered allows students to provide "peer review" and group solutions to clinical challenges. Students need to take an active part in their evaluations through the completion of written self-evaluation as well as peer evaluation for group activities. This self-evaluation begins with a written self-assessment (as part of the portfolio development) and continues throughout the course during individual conferences and through journaling.

Written journals and logs should not be a mere listing of activities but should synthesize content from other courses and demonstrate its application. Students can be given specific writing assignments such as the exploration of an issue or a response to a clinical scenario. The instructor can assign half of the clinical group to take one side of an organizational or clinical issue and the other group to the opposing view. Students can present and discuss their views later in clinical conference.

Nursing care plans can explore in-depth a particular client or family health problem. They are not the traditional care plan used in acute-care settings but are adapted to the setting and types of clients encountered, such as a patient teaching plan for an individual without a support system. Standardized care plans should be avoided except as background sources.

Novice students need opportunities to review their interactions with clients to refine their therapeutic communication skills. Process recordings may be valuable especially in situations where the opportunities for the instructor to accompany the student are limited. The instructor reviews the process recording for both content and communication process, as well as the student's evaluation of communication techniques (Fontaine & Fletcher 1999). If confidentiality permits, tape recording or videotaping can be very useful in recording the interactions between students and clients. When students visit homes in pairs, the student acting as the recorder could videotape the student with primary responsibility for the visit. The students can select what they anticipate will be the most salient portion of the exchange to present to the instructor. They should also share their rationale for their selections.

Student-developed products such as pamphlets, brochures, and case studies are additional ways to determine how the student is progressing in meeting the course objectives. In our community-based nursing course, each clinical group develops a case study that the group believes is representative of the population served by its clinical agency (Box 6–2). The group then shares its case studies so that all groups have a sense of the clients served across the clinical sites.

Because the clinical groups are in a variety of settings, our clinical instructors who teach the community-based course came to a consensus on critical behaviors and criteria for accomplishing those behaviors. Each semester the

Box 6-2 Learning Exercise for Faculty Use

Critical Behaviors

Think about the critical behaviors that you want students to develop in a specific setting. Make a list of criteria you would use to assess these behaviors in students. You might want to include in your list criteria for students to use in peer evaluation.

---

faculty discusses clinical activities that can be done repeatedly so that growth can be demonstrated over time versus those that are only available once and should be evaluated more on preparation and thinking through actions, rather than actual skill. There are also skills that may be repetitious of previous clinicals but demand new critical-thinking skills. For example, checking blood pressures in a walk-in clinic is different from assessing morning vital signs on a medical-surgical unit in an acute-care setting. In a community-based setting, the student needs to consider when to refer and to whom to refer in relation to a high blood pressure reading. Similarly, when a student is working in an immunization clinic, he or she may have previous experience with administering intramuscular and subcutaneous injections, but be unfamiliar with childhood immunization schedules and how to evaluate interruptions in that schedule. Handling these types of situations requires critical-thinking skills that will need to be reflected in the clinical evaluation process in community-based settings.

Because students often work in pairs to accomplish home visits or in small groups to develop health education materials and sessions, they need to participate in providing and receiving peer evaluation. The clinical instructor should assist the students in establishing evaluation criteria and methods for delivering the evaluation so that students consider the overall process, content, and outcomes. It is often helpful to begin with a question such as, "If you were to work together again, what would you do differently next time?" Successful experiences with peer evaluation are essential in preparing undergraduate nursing students for the collaborative practice that they will be expected to enter after graduation.

In the following example, we will look at what can happen when a student has difficulty performing in a community-based clinical rotation and how the use of a contract between the instructor and student can be helpful in resolving the problem.

When a Student Is in Jeopardy

Almost from the beginning of the semester, Hilary had difficulty performing at the expected level of competency for a novice nursing student. She was often late for the clinical day because of her long commute through inconsistent traffic patterns. She often procrastinated and would get to the end of the week (second clinical day) without having made a home visit to any of the three families assigned to her. She would state that no one answered the phone, but she had really only attempted to call once in the late afternoon. By the fourth week of clinical, she was behind in the health education materials that she had promised to prepare for use in teaching safety to elementary school students. Her peers were also complaining that she had not contributed her share to the group community assessment. Her weekly journal entries were usually submitted late and contained only brief references to attempts to complete activities and excuses as to why they were not done.

It was clear that we could not wait for a mid-term evaluation conference to clarify expectations and get Hilary back on track for successful completion of her community-based clinical nursing course. We sat down together for a private "contracting" session. We began by reviewing the course objectives and the practical aspects of accomplishing them through the clinical activities available in this agency. We then assigned completion dates to the tasks so that she would have endpoints in mind as she structured each clinical day.

As the contract developed, Hilary began to see the need for daily and weekly objectives that could be modified based on developments each day, as well as for a long-term plan for accomplishment of major projects by the end of the semester. Hilary shared her apprehensions surrounding the environment and some of the less structured aspects of the clinical rotation. We were then able to agree on what she could do independently, and what assistance she needed from me. She had been reluctant to share her apprehensions with me, for fear of jeopardizing her grade. Our "contracting" session helped her to understand the real dangers of procrastination and avoidance of the problem areas (Table 6–4).

Table 6-4

George Mason University College of Nursing and Health Science
Shared Responsibilities of Student and Faculty for Students in Clinical/Academic Jeopardy

FACULTY MEMBER WILL DRAW UP WRITTEN CONTRACT WITH THE STUDENT STATING SPECIFICALLY WHAT MUST BE DONE TO IMPROVE WEAK AREAS.

Hilary will be on time for clinical every day.

Hilary will participate in each clinical conference (weekly on Thursday afternoons).

Hilary will consult with field nurse for suggestions as to the best time to contact each family (to be accomplished by end of next clinical day).

Hilary will have a list of health-education materials needed for safety teaching (to be accomplished by end of first clinical day next week).

Hilary will attend clinical group meeting this afternoon and make a list of her responsibilities for the group community assessment.

Hilary will submit weekly journal entry for instructor's review and suggestions at the end of each clinical week.

THE CONTRACT WILL INCLUDE STUDENT RESPONSIBILITIES AND ROLE OF FACULTY AS CO-PARTNER IN STATED OUTCOMES, TO ACHIEVE SATISFACTORY STANDING IN COURSE.

The instructor will accompany Hilary on first visit to each of the families to assist in assessing the family's needs and establishing objective.

Hilary will develop objectives and evaluation criteria for each home visit with the instructor prior to each visit.

The instructor will review the health education materials and make suggestions as needed.

Hilary will participate in peer review regarding her work on the community assessment.

The instructor will meet with Hilary weekly for the next 3 weeks to review this contract and discuss progress and needed modifications.

As part of the weekly conference, Hilary will note on the clinical evaluation tool, the areas where she has made progress.

At the midterm evaluation conference, Hilary will have objectives for the remainder of the semester and will have activities in mind to accomplish those objectives.

Student Signature: _____ Instructor Signature: _____

Date: _____

Other Forms of Evaluation

In addition to participating in self-evaluation, students also in take part in ongoing course and clinical agency evaluation. In our program, students complete "course evaluation forms" (Table 6–5), as well as "clinical agency evaluation forms" (Table 6–6).

Completion of these forms provides students with the opportunity to evaluate the facility as a site for the course and to evaluate the instructor's teaching methods. The course coordinator reviews the course evaluation forms and prepares a summary (Table 6–7). The summary is shared at the final course meeting when the semester is evaluated, and recommendations are made for revising or improving the course. The clinical placement coordinator receives and summarizes the students' clinical agency evaluation forms as well as those completed by each clinical instructor (Table 6–8).

Many community-based agencies are small with very tight budgets, and they may be in a constant state of flux in terms of ownership, leadership, financing, and services offered. Opportunities for student experiences may change drastically from semester to semester. Therefore, it is imperative to maintain written evaluations of the sites from both the student and instructor perspectives. Because our junior level community-based clinical

---

Table 6-5

George Mason University College of Nursing and Health Science
Clinical Course Evaluation Tool

This evaluation is for Course ___ Section ___ Semester ___ Year ___

Directions: Please assist in evaluating this course by writing a brief narrative response to each of the following questions. Return this evaluation in the enclosed envelope to the course coordinator.

Is this clinical setting a good placement for student learning and why?

Were the course objectives realistic and how could they be improved?

My instructor did the following things well related to this clinical.

My instructor could improve in the following areas relative to this clinical.

Use back of sheet if necessary. You need not sign your name. Thank you for your comments.

Table 6-6

George Mason University College of Nursing and Health Science
Student Evaluation of Clinical Agency

AGENCY: _____   **SEMESTER/YEAR:** _____

FACULTY: _____   **COURSE:** _____

How are the course objectives met in this clinical agency?

What are the strengths of this clinical site?

What are the challenges that you encountered at this clinical site?

Suggestions to improve your learning at this clinical agency:

Please return this form to the Clinical Placement Coordinator.

---

course is offered only in the spring semester each academic year, the clinical placement coordinator needs the clinical agency evaluations when he or she begins planning early in the fall semester for the spring community-based clinical sites. The placement coordinator is also responsible for eliciting feedback from the agency staff regarding their satisfaction with the experience.

CHALLENGES AND REWARDS OF UNSTRUCTURED CLINICAL SETTINGS

Much of what is reported in the literature regarding clinical faculty workload issues is concerned with acute-care clinical rather than community-based settings (Oermann MH 1994,1998; Oermann & Standfest 1997; Schuster, et al. 1997). Despite many years of clinical practice and teaching experience in acute-care settings, faculty often feel like novices when they work with students in community-based agencies (Tagliareni & Murray 1995). Clinical instructors supervising students in community-based settings may often feel that they have overwhelming responsibilities, especially at the beginning of the semester. One of our clinical instructors described it in this way:

> *The semester began with a rocky start. I was new to the metropolitan area, to the university, and to the clinical agency. Although I have a strong theoretical and practice background in public health, I was not familiar with a community-based curriculum and the placement of junior level*

Table 6-7

George Mason University College of Nursing and Health Science
Course Report Form (CRF)

(To be used by course coordinators)

Directions: At the end of semester when all Executive Summaries for the course have been collected, make a composite report, using this form, to the program evaluation committee chair. Save the summaries for at least two semesters before discarding.

Course ____ Sections ____ Semester ____ Year ____

List of major issues discussed:

Possible courses of action:

Possible outcomes of actions listed:

Recommendations to curriculum committee:

Return to Chair, Program Evaluation Committee

---

students in public schools for clinical experiences. The students in my assigned clinical group, in turn, related concerns and uncertainties about their clinical sites.

Although I had many ideas and community connections for them to explore, the students had difficulty letting the semester "play out." They wanted to see the whole semester mapped out during the first week. I tried to show them that we would have to let the semester develop. Although the school's principal and her staff were very welcoming from the beginning, there were many variables to control: nursing students were ambivalent about the clinical, teachers were unclear as to the nursing students' role, a school nurse had expectations, children and parents had special needs. At times it was overwhelming . . .

Oermann (1998) reported that regardless of clinical setting, instructors cited adequate orientation to the clinical setting, supportive colleagues, and consistency in teaching assignments as most helpful in relieving their stress as clinical faculty.

Our experiences with seasoned faculty members moving into community-based clinical settings have mirrored Oermann's findings. Clinical instructors assigned to community-based settings need orientation time with each other to become familiar with course objectives, common threads of clinical experiences, suggested learning activities, and evaluation strategies, as well as orientation time within the clinical agency to

Table 6-8

George Mason University College of Nursing and Health Science
Clinical Agency Evaluation

INSTRUCTOR:	**AGENCY:**
COURSE NO.:	**UNIT(S) USED:**
FOR SEMESTER:	**IMMEDIATE POINT OF CONTACT PERSON:**
NO. STUDENTS SUPERVISED:	
TODAY'S DATE:	**PHONE NO. OF UNIT(S):**

Use the back of the form if necessary.

Short description of agency/unit(s):

Strengths:

Limitations:

Recommendations:

Please return completed form to _____ at the end of the semester.

which they are assigned. The course coordinator orchestrates the orientation to the course, whereas each clinical instructor arranges time in the clinical agency. Written materials, such as "Guidelines for Clinical Supervision in Undergraduate Practicum Courses" provided in Chapter 1 and "Shared Responsibilities of Student and Faculty" (see Table 6–4), are useful tools for instructors to have.

Faculty development opportunities prior to the beginning of the semester and throughout the semester are also quite helpful. The clinical instructors teaching our junior level community-based nursing course have varied backgrounds. All are either masters- or doctorally prepared with specialty preparation in community health nursing, maternity nursing, psychiatric nursing, pediatric nursing, or medical-surgical nursing. This diversity has greatly enriched our curriculum and our students' clinical learning experiences. Many of our faculty, however, have limited or no clinical experience outside acute-care settings. As we moved our clinicals out into the community, we discovered that the faculty needed some retraining or retooling. Areas most in need of faculty development included physical assessment (across the lifespan), neighborhood and community assessment, process of home visiting, principles of epidemiology, environmental health, and health education planning and implementation.

Faculty members need to familiarize themselves with the current thinking on the continuum of acute, community-based, and population-focused care so that they can assist their students in understanding these important concepts.

Participation in faculty development workshops also contributed to collegiality among the clinical instructors. Discussion of health-care issues within the context of the clinical experiences we are building for our students brings the faculty closer together. This type of discussion also assists faculty to think about particular clinical sites and how to tailor coursework to the site and its community members (Oneha, et al. 1998). Monthly course meetings continue the dialogue begun during the orientation period and provide ongoing support to the clinical instructors as they become more familiar with the course, the clinical site, and their students. As one instructor commented:

The monthly meetings with everyone teaching the course, as well as my occasional conversations throughout the semester with the course coordinator and clinical placement coordinator, were very helpful to me. These contacts helped me to feel less isolated and to maintain my focus on student learning and the needs of the community we serve.

Whenever possible, it is important for faculty to have the opportunity to return to the same clinical site more than once to build a continuity network of experiences and mentors for the students and to develop a sense of accomplishment in their work. Many of our faculty members report feeling much more successful during the second semester in a clinical site than during the first:

It's very satisfying to return to the same clinical site for a second semester! What a big difference—staff nurses come looking for students offering new experiences and volunteer to accompany them on home visits for "Healthy Family" assessments or on a nursing home admissions workup.

Additionally, the clinical placement coordinator hears from clinical agency personnel that they prefer consistency in clinical instructor from semester to semester. Not only is the burden of orientation lessened, but also is the value of partnering with an instructor over several semesters apparent to the staff. A clinical instructor with experience in the agency knows policies, personnel, and clients, and can build from previous experiences instead of beginning again.

Despite the many challenges of being a clinical instructor in an unstructured, community-based clinical setting, our clinical instructors report a great deal of satisfaction with their experiences. They enjoy the opportunity to demonstrate to health-care professionals the value of having nursing students as part of the team.

For me, this was an exciting teaching experience because it offered a new opportunity to work in a multidisciplinary context while providing comprehensive care to children from 0 to 3 years old with special needs. It was totally up to me to approach the staff and set up the clinical experiences for my students. At first it was difficult to establish the

nursing role because the staff had never worked with nurses before. I met regularly with the co-directors as well as the individual therapists in PT, Speech, and OT to assure the networks of communication.

During the semester, the staff came to acknowledge nursing's contributions in coordinating and providing continuity of care in the home. As they realized that nursing students could provide services to their clients, staff members sought out the nursing students and referred clients to them. The nursing students were able to make many home visits to reinforce and enhance behaviors presented during therapy sessions. Several of the families requested continued services from the students and felt we made a difference in their lives.

Students often come to the community-based clinical uncertain about the value of the experience and unsure of their ability to perform adequately. The faculty also enjoy watching their students grow and change.

There are usually one or two students in each group who are not pleased to be in a community-based setting instead of an acute-care setting. It is very satisfying to see them find their "niche" in the community through their teaching activities. I remember one particular student who was not pleased on the first day of clinical when she learned that there was no set agenda for each clinical day of the semester. She was assigned to an excellent staff nurse and became involved in working with children with special needs and disabilities. By the end of the semester, this student had decided that community health was her chosen field and that she would apply for a job when she graduated.

Previously in the chapter, we discussed the concept of faculty partnering with students to provide nursing care. Although faculty are at first uncertain about this and wonder how to separate "teaching" and "evaluation," they are often quite pleased with the results of their efforts.

My main objective with my clinical students for this community-based experience was cultivating the essence of CARING. I saw this through the work of one student assigned to a fourth- and fifth-grade class of MR students. She observed the students at lunch after spending the morning listening to their descriptions of their tummy aches. She then shared with me her ideas for a teaching activity related to nutrition.

She began by conducting a needs assessment of her target group. Using a very simple questionnaire that she designed, she engaged the students in a 24-hour recall and a daily log that covered 3 additional days. She constructed graphs and pie charts as she analyzed her data. With the children, she taught the food pyramid, went grocery shopping as a field trip, and made a healthy lunch with them. She presented her findings to the school public health nurse, the principal, and the clinic room aide. This resulted in a stronger commitment to sound nutrition for this special group of children. The student demonstrated her commitment to the children. Her work reflected critical thinking beyond the scope of practice for a junior level nursing student, and it was laced with caring.

The most rewarding part of the experience comes at the end of the semester when students present their teaching plans and other activities for clients and staff members. At this time, the students' relationships with clients and staff reflect both the personal and professional growth that occurred throughout the semester. Students' comfort in the setting and awareness of their contributions both to the clients and to the staff mirror their level of investment and commitment throughout the semester.

References

American Association of Colleges of Nursing (1999). Essential clinical resources for nursing's academic mission. Washington, DC: American Association of Colleges of Nursing.

Baillie, L (1993). Factors affecting student nurses' learning in community placements: A phenomenological study. J Adv Nurs 18, 1043–1053.

Carroll, MC, et al. (1999). Assessing students' perceived threats to safety in the community: Instrument refinement. Nurs Educ 24, 31–35.

DeLaGarza, S, & Martinez-Rogers, N (1998). Community clinical sites for psychiatric nursing students. J Nurs Educ 37(3), 142–143.

Faller, HS, et al. (1995). Bridge to the future: Nontraditional clinical settings, concepts and issues. J Nurs Educ 34, 344–349.

Fontaine, KL & Fletcher, JS (1999). Mental health nursing, 4 ed. Menlo Park, CA: Addison Wesley Longman, Inc.

Ford-Gilboe, M, et al. (1997). The effect of a clinical practicum on undergraduate nursing students' self-efficacy for community-based family nursing practice. J Nurs Educ 36(5), 212–219.

Hayes, ER, et al. (1996). Managing fear associated with nursing in urban environments: First steps. Public Health Nurs 13, 90–96.

Herrman, J, et al. (1998). Beyond hospital walls: Educating pediatric nurses for the next millennium. Pediatr Nurs 24, 96-99.

Lindemann, CA (1989). Clinical teaching: Paradoxes and paradigms. In National League for Nursing. Curriculum revolution: Reconceptualizing nursing education. New York: National League for Nursing.

Oermann, MH (1994). Professional nursing education in the future: Changes and challenges. J Obstet Gynecol Neonatal Nurs 23(2), 153-159.

Oermann, MH (1998). Role strain of clinical faculty. J Prof Nurs 14(6), 329-334.

Oermann, MH, & Standfest, KM (1997). Differences in stress and challenge in clinical practice among ADN and BSN students in varying clinical courses. J Nurs Educ 36(5), 228-233.

Oneha, MF, et al. (1998). Ensuring quality nursing education in community-based settings. Nurse Educ 23, 26-31.

O'Neil, ES, & Pennington, EA (1996). Preparing acute care nurses for community-based care. N HC Perspect Community 17(2), 62-65.

Palmer, NS (1995). Moving student clinical experiences into primary care settings. Nurs Educ 20(4), 12-14.

Schuster, P, et al. (1997). Workload issues in clinical nursing education. J Prof Nurs 13(3), 154-159.

Tagliareni, ME, & Murray, J (1995). Community-focused experiences in the associate degree nursing curriculum. J Nurs Educ 34, 366-371.

SECTION 2

Faculty Application in Community-based Sites

CHAPTER 7

Teaching Students in a Senior Center

Joanne C. Langan

Learning Objectives

1) List key attributes that faculty members need to teach effectively in a community-based senior center.
2) Discuss the challenges in establishing a community-based site in a senior center.
3) Specify strategies that facilitate acceptance of faculty and students in a community-based site.
4) Discuss faculty supervision and student accountability in a community-based site.
5) Identify health-promotion activities that can be performed in a senior center to enhance student learning.

This chapter discusses what I believe to be essential qualities of a faculty member to teach effectively in a community-based site. The senior center is the specific clinical site and includes the participants in the adult day care and the residents in the assisted living section of the same building. I also share the story of my experience in developing the senior center as a clinical site.

As most nursing faculty members know, changes in the health-care system require more community-focused experiences for nursing students. Yoder and colleagues (1997) describe their experience in developing successful home-health clinical experiences for students early in the curriculum. At George Mason University's (GMU) College of Nursing and Health Science, community-based experiences are begun early in the nursing curriculum as well. All nursing courses are taught during the baccalaureate nursing student's junior and senior years. The first community-based course is taught in the second semester of the junior year and emphasizes individuals, families, and small groups. The senior-year community experience focuses on populations. This chapter focuses on the junior-year experience.

Perhaps the greatest attributes a faculty member can possess in teaching a community-based clinical are communication skills, knowledge, flexibility and energy, creativity, love of teaching and learning, and appreciation for the community. Because the idea of nursing students and faculty members practicing in community-based sites is a novel concept to some agencies, the idea must be explained and often "sold" to the community site. The faculty member must be able to communicate expectations and responsibilities to agency administrators and staff, the health-care team, students, individual clients, families, and groups. Each of these entities has specific needs for information on varying frequencies. For instance, the communication between the faculty member and the agency administrator may be periodic, whereas the communication with the students will be constant.

Knowledge about the individuals, families, and groups you and your students will be working with is also important. One must be familiar with the resources available to these individuals at the agency level, in the community, and on the broader governmental or political level. Ideally, the faculty member would have some faculty practice experience with the clinical agency where students are supervised or have previously worked with similar kinds of clients. Although faculty practice outside of the teacher's role with students is not a requirement in most instances, it enhances teaching effectiveness and offers credibility with the agency. If the faculty member has not had recent experience with the individuals and groups assigned, I suggest a great deal of reading, visiting the agency and its affiliates, and networking among resource services. I did not have previous experience working at the senior center, but because I had prior and recent experience with the geriatric population, I was very comfortable. I read extensively and used current articles and materials addressing issues of interest to the geriatric population in my teaching. I networked with agency personnel who supported this population in the community. It was important to be familiar with community course offerings and support groups for caregivers such as those offered by the Alzheimer's Association.

Flexibility and energy are mentioned together because of the great deal of energy required to remain flexible. Although the acute-care facilities have relatively stable tasks and activities, the community settings are variable. Individuals and families do not necessarily present at the community sites with regularity. However, the senior center participants attended at regular intervals unless they were ill, took family trips, or their family members were unable to transport them. Even the best preparation and planning did not matter if the clients did not come to the senior center or the activities schedule had changed.

Students prepared mini-teaching projects and blood pressure, hearing, and vision screenings. At times, they were discouraged if their planned events were poorly attended. Together, the students and I would discuss the situations, engage in some critical thinking, and work on "Plan B." I emphasized flexibility, which I consider an essential trait for all nurses. This flexibility does require a great deal of energy because the faculty member must consider all factors such as the students, the clients, the agency, scheduling, and course objectives. "Changing gears" in student activities must have the goal of enhancing student learning, not just filling a gap in time.

Because no two community clinical sites are alike, the faculty members are often required to be creative in their teaching approach and in designing student experiences.

One set of course objectives are met in 12 different community-based sites (Table 7–1).

I developed a list of sample activities that are unique to the senior center that students may perform to achieve credit for each of the 10 clinical objectives and behaviors. Table 7–2 is an example of a course objective and suggested activities that would fit the objective.

I verbally explain and give students copies of the suggested activities that would fit each of the 10 objectives. The student responses may take place in clinical preconference or postconference, or may appear in the students' journals that are submitted weekly. Again, the creativity is important in meeting the needs of individual students and clients.

Next, clinical faculty need to possess a love of teaching and learning. At times, the faculty members are the only nurses in the community settings. They must model appropriate nursing behaviors for nursing students. In the acute-care setting, faculty members may find themselves relying on staff nurses to assist in teaching technologies

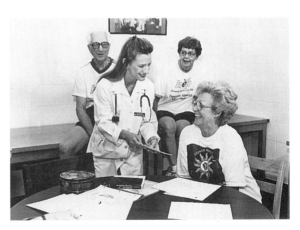

Table 7-1

George Mason University College of Nursing and Health Science
Nursing as a Health Service I
4 credits—clinical

COURSE OBJECTIVES:

Upon completion of this course the student will be able to:

1. Incorporate concepts from pathophysiology, health assessment, and other technologies into the nursing process.
2. Develop therapeutic relationships with individuals and their families.
3. Incorporate knowledge of epidemiology, health patterns, and cultural diversity to determine needs of individuals, families, and small groups.
4. Collaborate with individuals, families, and members of the health team to determine health education needs.
5. Demonstrate caring and sensitive nursing interventions for individuals and their families who are experiencing developmental and situational crises.
6. Anticipate the need for health-care coordination and continuity of care.
7. Perform selected technologies in a variety of settings.
8. Demonstrate professional behaviors.
9. Demonstrate accountability for time management in the community-based care of individuals, families, and small groups.
10. Plan and implement health-promotion and disease-prevention strategies with individuals, families, and small groups.

and nursing skills. This luxury is seldom found in the community. Often, there are multiple opportunities for the faculty member to teach students, clients, and agency staff. Conversely, faculty members may be afforded the opportunity to learn from agency personnel and clients. Students and agency staff are very perceptive to the faculty's willingness to teach and enthusiasm for learning.

Finally, faculty members who teach in the community must have a true appreciation for the community as a place to teach and for the community of individuals, families, and small groups. Our community site was located in a lovely setting with a myriad of support systems and resources. The vulnerable population was the aged, and there was a great deal of cultural diversity among the clients. This rich tapestry of cultural differences enhanced the student experiences. We were also able to discuss cultural differences between the youthful nursing

Table 7-2

Sample Activities

COURSE OBJECTIVE #1:

Incorporate concepts from pathophysiology, health assessment, and other technologies into the nursing process.

SUGGESTED ACTIVITIES:

Discuss the pathophysiology of the client and family members with a description of expected behaviors, medications, activities, and limitations. Include your health assessment findings, vital signs, and observed behaviors. Is there a match between expected and actual behaviors?

students and the elderly clients. Anderson and colleagues (1996) warn that policy makers and the media tend to erroneously consider the elderly as a homogeneous group. We all gained a renewed appreciation for the geriatric population who helped to dispel a number of myths that Rowe and Kahn (1999) discussed about aging—that to be old is to be sick, and that you can't teach an old dog new tricks (p 12). Many of the participants in the senior center had no or minimal disability and learned new information well. They were enjoyable, and some were even vigorous. One student shared the following:

> I really had fun at the party. I danced with several of the chair-bound participants, which they seemed to appreciate. They sat, and I held their hands and danced. I danced with J.P. who almost killed me. She is strong and energetic. She held on to me so tight and tossed me around the dance floor. She was singing the whole time and I was laughing. It was really fun.

As the instructor, I freely shared my appreciation for the community setting at the senior center and my appreciation for the opportunity to work with these clients.

HISTORY OF DEVELOPING THE SENIOR CENTER AS A CLINICAL SITE

In the fall of 1997, I was in the administrative faculty role of Clinical Placement Coordinator and Community Liaison. In this role, I continually had my "radar" out for potential clinical sites for our undergraduate nursing program. Competition for clinical sites was an issue for acute-care experiences, but even more difficult for community-based experiences. In part, the difficulty was because of changes in agency populations, agency administrators, and the need to place up to 10 students in one clinical section. Many community agencies are small and cannot physically accommodate 10 students and a faculty member. Because change is a constant, the networking to locate potential sites needs to be constant.

Informal discussion with those knowledgeable with the site and course objectives is a good first step in developing a site for student placement. Informal discussions can lead to further investigation of a potential site or convince the clinical placement coordinator to proceed no further.

In the same fall semester, I had an informal discussion with a colleague about an enthusiastic nurse who was a co-director of an adult day-care center. This community nurse was a guest speaker to undergraduate nursing students in my colleague's class. My fellow faculty member convinced me to call the nurse and visit the senior center. I knew I was about to embark on an adventure and a number of challenges. As Yoder and colleagues (1997) state, "There is never an ideal time to organize an innovative new student clinical experience" (p 494).

I called the nurse at the agency and explained the referral. I immediately mentioned the key requirements of our community-based clinical experience. I explained that we would be working with individuals, families, and small groups and would concentrate on health promotion and disease prevention in vulnerable populations. This information was received very positively, and I was invited to tour the facility.

One of our first tasks was to review the course syllabus, objectives, and required activities together. We discussed each requirement and how each could be met. The co-director was able to suggest a number of activities to fulfill course objectives.

As we toured the facility, I remained cognizant of the course objectives and tried to visualize 10 students and an instructor in the center. Because the adult day-care center had an average of 30 to 40 participants each weekday, we did not feel that the space could accommodate 10 students. The assisted living "home" was directly one floor above the adult day-care center. Assisted living residents frequently joined the day-care participants for activities. Dividing the 10 students between these two floors seemed to be a logical solution.

Another very important element in this initial visit was the affiliation agreement or contract discussion. The adult day-care co-director needed to share the contract with the agency administrator because she did not have signature authority. I explained each section of the contract to her and offered to do the same with the administrator. The fully executed contract is a requirement before students may begin the clinical rotation at each site.

I did not know at the time the contract was being negotiated that I would be the faculty member who would be taking students to this particular clinical site. The contract was fully executed and on file at both the university and at the agency. I chose to become a half-time faculty member and was assigned to the senior center. Of course I was delighted with my assignment because I had met many of the staff at the center and was pleased with their mission and philosophy. I was ready to begin planning for this new site weeks in advance of the spring 1998 semester.

Letters of Introduction

One of the course objectives for our junior-level community clinical was the completion of a family assessment. To facilitate the identification of one family for each of the 10 students, I chose to send a letter of introduction to each family of the adult day-care participants (Table 7–3). These letters contained a brief description of the clinical course, the purpose of the student and faculty presence, a list of options for services, and a request for participation.

Another letter asked for volunteers for family assessments and to receive the students during home visits although home visits were not required for the course (Table 7–4).

The associate dean of undergraduate programs reviewed and approved the communications before they were sent. As a courtesy to the agency, I asked the day-care co-director to review the letters. The agency offered to include the letters in their regular mailings.

Planning Student Activities

An orientation day was planned for the students on campus to introduce the course, the syllabus, and the requirements. Similarly, an orientation was planned for the first day in the agency. The students met the administrators, staff, and participants in the adult day-care center and the residents in the assisted living unit.

Perhaps the greatest challenge of the orientation (and semester) was to assist the students in acclimating to an unstructured setting. One of the purposes of a senior center is to provide a safe environment for loved ones while family members must be away from the home and go to work. The participants are typically dropped off in the morning before the commute to work and are picked up after the workday. The residents in the assisted living area are already "at home." Although this community's residents generally maintained a routine schedule, some participants had varied schedules of attendance. Unlike the acute-care or long-term care settings, this community setting did not offer the rigidity of a strict schedule. From the students' perspective, this lack of structure also meant a lack of security.

We needed to plan activities collaboratively with the agency. Students were anxious to achieve their family assessments, therapeutic communication recordings, and teaching projects but needed to be cognizant of the needs of the individual clients and their families. The participants and residents were actively engaged in a myriad of activities from singing, dancing, and bowling to trips to the "on-campus" beauty shop.

Assigning individual clients, families, and home visits was an easy task once the family responses to the letter of introduction were received. Some students bonded with particular clients immediately and requested those clients and their families. Other families were chosen randomly. As the entire clinical group became familiar with the participants and clients, students began to brainstorm ideas for fun activities (rapport-builders, mini-teaching projects, and the major teaching projects).

Even though home visits were not required, those students who were invited to the clients' homes were grateful for the experience. Some families chose to complete the family assessments with the students in a quiet area of the day-care center, whereas some families chose to

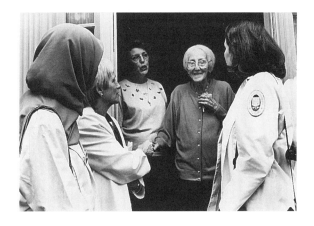

Table 7-3

Letter of Introduction

George Mason University
4400 University Drive
Fairfax, VA. 22030
(703) 993-1000
TDD: (703) 993-1002

December 8, 1999

Dear Health-care Center Families:

Beginning January 23, 1999, 10 George Mason University nursing students and their instructor will spend Wednesdays and Fridays at the Health-care Center. The focus of the students' clinical course is the health assessment of individuals and families in ambulatory and assisted living settings. The students will teach clients, families, and staff about health promotion and disease prevention. The following is a list of possible activities students may perform. If you are interested in participating in our program through a home visit or would like to have your family member included in the activities, please place a check next to the activity and sign below. The faculty member will contact you. All activities and services are free.

If you have any question, please call the instructor at 703-993-1902. The last clinical day of the semester is May 1, 2000.

Thank you!

Joanne C. Langan, RN, MSN

Instructor

George Mason University, College of Nursing and Health Science
Spring, 2000 Clinical Activities

_____	Health Education Project (Individual or Family)	_____	Nutrition Assessment & Counseling
_____	Health & Wellness Assessment	_____	Exercise Programs
_____	Mini-Screening (Blood Pressure)	_____	Mini–Mental Status Exam
_____	Health Fair in Agency	_____	Identification of Community Resources
_____	Home Visiting for Family Assessments & Health Education	_____	Identification of Resources for Obtaining Medical Supplies
_____	Assessment of Safety of Environment (Home/Work/Play)	_____	Medication Review and Education for Compliance
		_____	Assistance with Activities of Daily Living (ADLs)

(Modifications necessary due to mobility problems or chronic illness)

_____
Signature and Date

Please return this form to the Health-care Center in the GMU CNHS return folder.

Table 7-4

Family Letter

January 20, 2000

Dear Health-care Center Families:

We are delighted that we have the opportunity to work with your loved ones in the day-care and assisted living settings once again. The 10 junior nursing students and I will be presenting several mini-teaching projects focusing on health promotion and disease prevention. We will provide blood pressure screenings each Wednesday and Friday from February 3 through May 7, 2000.

The students are required to complete a family assessment as one of the course objectives. The family assessment consists of an interview with a family member or members to discuss such topics as family composition and medical, dental, and nutritional health and concerns. The students are practicing assessment and health interview skills as well as determining if there are any services or resources that they can provide the families. The interviews may take place at the Center at the family's convenience.

We would like to "match" 10 families with the 10 students. You are under no obligation to participate and may withdraw your name at any time. All information is kept confidential.

Thank you for your willingness to provide learning opportunities for these nursing students.

Sincerely,

Joanne C. Langan, RN, PhD

Assistant Professor

(703) 993-1902

Yes, the nursing student may call to arrange an appointment to meet with me.

Name_____ Date_____ Phone_____

Best time to reach me:

Signature_____ Participant/Resident Name_____

(Please return this form to the Health-care Center by February 17)

---

talk with the students before or after a visit with their loved ones in their resident "homes" in assisted living. A serendipitous finding of the majority of students was the opportunity for therapeutic communication sessions with the families. The students felt greatly rewarded that they were able to be with the family members and listen to the expression of grief and loss as the participants or residents experienced alterations in mental and physical function.

Accounting for Student Time

Students were held accountable for their own clinical time. We calculated that a minimum of 196 hours of clinical time was required for the course. Each student kept his or her own time log and documented each clinical day's activities and time spent. Not all of the time needed to be spent at the clinical agency. We typically had preconferences and postconferences in the senior center's conference room. However, students were free to visit other community agencies to secure pamphlets and information pertinent to the care of their clients and families, for example. A list of acceptable alternative activities outside of the clinical agency is in Table 7–5.

If a student wanted to plan an alternative experience, the student was required to discuss the plan with the faculty member prior to the day of the alternative experience. GMU's College of Nursing and Health Science provides a form that the student and faculty member complete prior to the student's alternative experience or visit. The form encourages the student to formulate objectives for the experience and to identify a responsible person at the agency with whom the faculty member can communicate if necessary. This requirement for a contact person at the alternative agency is a very important link to fulfill the responsibility of faculty supervision.

Table 7-5

Community Activities/Experiences Outside of Agency

Visits to community agencies for resources

Visits to library to search Internet for resources

Home visits

Visits to day-care programs

Visits to assisted living facilities

Visits to long-term care/transition facilities

Hospital visits to see hospitalized clients

Visits to medical supply stores to compare prices for assistive devices for the home

Visits to physician and dental offices to discuss special needs of the elderly

Attendance at conferences/in-services on topics relevant to elderly clients or family issues (Alzheimer's support group, the family caregiver, choosing appropriate placement for elderly parents)

Faculty Supervision and Communication Strategies

All faculty members are responsible for the supervision of students during clinical experiences. It is ideal that faculty members be physically present with the students. However, the faculty member may be away from the clinical agency with a student or students on home visits. In the latter case, the faculty member must be accessible to the students and agency by pager. The clinical agency must be comfortable with the arrangement and name a nurse or responsible professional with whom the students may confer in the faculty member's absence. We posted a student assignment sheet in a prominent place in the agency. Agency staff members were able to tell, at a glance, where each student was for the day and the next week.

At the senior center, I was easily accessible to the students in both the day-care center and in the assisted living unit. I wore the pager at all times in case the students, agency, or college needed to reach me. Another communication strategy was to elicit feedback from the senior center administrator, co-directors, and staff concerning the conduct of our clinical experience. They were very candid about positive and negative impressions of the students and me and offered suggestions. Conversely, they invited suggestions from the students and me regarding the clients, families, activities, and care plans.

Another key link in the communication chain is the family member of the participant or resident in the senior center. Family members were most accessible when they dropped off or picked up their loved ones. We were able to assess priority family issues and concerns and work on planning strategies to improve them. One of the family members voiced concern about her mother's wheelchair brakes during a visit with a nursing student. The student followed up on the complaint with the agency, found a person to repair the brakes, and the issue was resolved. Some of the family members were very tired and stressed by their own nuclear families and jobs so they were unable to seek the necessary resources. The families were very grateful for the attention and solutions offered by the students, and the students were pleased that they were able to make a difference in the clients' lives.

One of the areas that I failed to clarify early in the semester was the transportation of clients in wheelchairs.

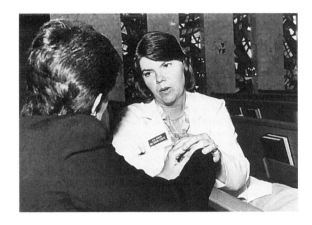

The agency policy was to take clients backwards on any downhill slope. I did not know of this policy and questioned why some personnel were transporting in that manner. The students and I were gently reminded that this method was the agency policy. We were asked to transport in this way to ensure client safety. We complied with the request but could have avoided an uncomfortable situation with better communication. This communication was also very important in distinguishing the students' scope of practice from other agency personnel.

Student Scope of Practice and Technologies and Services Offered

It was essential to communicate specific learning experiences and nursing student practice activities that would be expected of the students. Although the students were capable of assisting the participants and residents in performing activities of daily living and changing incontinent briefs, I emphasized that this was not the purpose of this community clinical. Emphasis was placed on health promotion, disease-prevention strategies through teaching, problem solving, and therapeutic communication. The students were not allowed to practice registered nurse activities without my direct supervision. However, the students eagerly anticipated the performance of new technologies, especially medication administration.

Junior-level nursing students are enrolled in a didactic community-based nursing course and an intermediate technologies course concurrently with the community-based clinical course. The laboratory technologies include sterile technique and medication administration via all routes. Senior citizens commonly take multiple medications and lack knowledge about proper administration and side effects. Nursing students often learn pharmacology in the classroom with no opportunity to apply the knowledge as it is learned (Wissmann & Wilmoth 1996). This is the case in many of the community-based sites. Our GMU nursing students typically take the pharmacology course during the same semester as the community clinical with no opportunity to apply the newly acquired knowledge and skills.

A very unique feature of this clinical site is the ability of the instructor to offer medication administration opportunities to the students. The students, under the instructor's supervision, administered all but intravenous medications. This activity gave the students opportunities to teach the participants and residents about their medications and health conditions. Concepts learned in

Table 7-6

Technologies/Services Offered in the Agency/Home

Health education project (individual, family, or small groups)

Health and wellness assessment

Mini-screening days (blood pressure)

Health fair in agency

Home visiting for family assessments and health education

Assessment of safety of environment (home/work/play)

Nutrition assessment and counseling

Exercise programs

Mini–Mental Status Exam

Identification of community resources

Identification of resources for obtaining medical supplies

Medication review and education for compliance

Assistance with activities of daily living (ADLs) (modifications necessary because of mobility problems or chronic illness)

their pharmacology course were reinforced and practiced. Medication administration at the adult day-care center and the assisted living unit simulated what the nurse might do on home visits with clients. The home-care or community-based clinical placement provides an opportunity for students to apply the theoretical knowledge and skills they obtained in the classroom and laboratory (Yoder, et al. 1997).

A list of technologies and services offered in the agencies and the homes is found in Table 7–6. Students appreciated the experience as a means to build confidence in their skills and to be better prepared for their next clinical experience in the acute-care setting.

Learning Experiences and Teaching Strategies

As already discussed, the students were expected to perform the outlined clinical behaviors to a satisfactory level. They were to conduct and report a family assessment using an assessment instrument such as the Family Health Protective Behaviors Assessment Tool (Kandzari & Howard 1981). Andresen and colleagues (1998) compared a variety of instruments to measure health-related quality of life and made recommendations for their use among community-living older adults. This type of tool might be an interesting addition to the type of tool we used at the senior center.

The family assessments could be conducted in the family home or in the senior center according to the family preference. From these assessments, the students were to prioritize nursing diagnoses and knowledge deficits. Health education projects were then developed as major teaching plans that each student would present to individuals, families, or small groups. Some students chose to present health-promotion, disease-prevention information to all three categories of audiences.

Three therapeutic communications were to be conducted, written, and analyzed according to therapeutic techniques employed or communication blocks used. Points were not deducted for communication blocks used. In fact, credit was given when blocks were identified and recognized. Students quickly learned that one of the most valued and effective of the therapeutic techniques is silence. The use of silence was difficult for

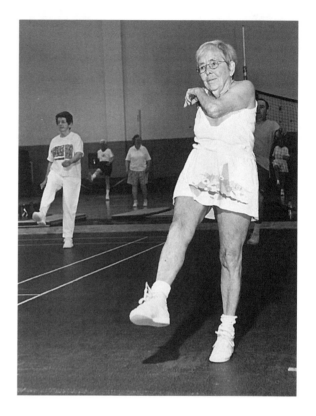

some to achieve because their anxiety during the conversation caused them to speak when they should have been listening.

Journals addressing each clinical day were submitted weekly. Journals were the only written materials submitted that were not graded. The faculty members felt that non-graded journals allowed students the freedom to express themselves freely and openly. However, I did ask the students to indicate and enumerate the clinical behaviors they achieved by marking the related clinical behavior objective numbers in the margins. By doing this, the students became very familiar with the behaviors on which they were being evaluated and became acutely aware of repetitive behaviors and those behaviors that were lacking in their performance.

Critical-thinking exercises were some of the most valued learning experiences. All 10 students were given case studies. They were asked to answer questions about the case using the nursing process and critical-thinking skills (Box 7–1). We had completed "practice" case studies in

| Box 7-1 | Learning Exercise for Faculty Use |

Critical Thinking Exercise

Mr. H has been staying with his daughter because of recent complications with radiation therapy for colon cancer. At first, he was very weak, fatigued, and had frequent bouts of diarrhea. Over the past few weeks, his strength has returned, and he is eating and feeling better but is still dizzy at times and unable to prepare his own meals. Mr. H is anxious to get back to his own home and also wants to resume driving his own car. In front of his daughter, he asks the nurse, "Why can't I start driving again?"

As the registered nurse, what is your response?

ASSESSMENT (Subjective and Objective Data)

List Problems:

Nursing Diagnosis:

(Of all the problems listed above, what is the priority problem?)

Write a three-part diagnosis.

Problem	Etiology	Signs and Symptoms
(Alterations in (Related To)	(As Evidenced By)	Client Health Status)

PLAN: Client Goals, Client Objectives (outcome criteria)

(Reverse the problem to a positive statement.)

Planning Nursing Orders: what the nurse will do to help the client meet the established client goals and objectives (i.e., assess, talk with, perform, turn, teach, instruct, consult, refer)

IMPLEMENTATION (i.e., observe response of client to care; then report, record, listen, instruct, administer, collect, perform, reinforce, discuss) _____

EVALUATE (Client goal achievement)

Client goal/objective achievement and resolution to the problem

Evaluate effectiveness of nursing orders

postconference throughout the semester. After a given time, the students located their classmate who had completed the same case study. Together, the partners were to evaluate what each had written and decide the best solutions to present to the class. The group continued to critique their own and others' work and to give the rationale for the favorable or negative critique. This proved to be an excellent culminating learning experience. A sample case study follows.

Table 7–5 is a list of activities outside the primary clinical agency assignment that the students could visit to enhance their learning during the community-based clinical. These visits culminated in a report presented to the clinical group describing the reason for the visit, the objectives achieved by the visit, the information learned, the materials gathered, and the way the learned information was used to teach health-promotion, disease-prevention strategies to our clients and their families at the senior center. One student successfully completed this exercise as follows: By visiting other senior centers in the area, she gathered information on resources for the elderly, including Area Agencies on Aging, federal agencies, area clearinghouses, nutrition services, and transportation services. She then compiled a resource book with all resource agency names, locations, and phone numbers. She taught our clinical group, her peers, how to use this resource book and share the information with their clients.

Table 7–6 is a list of technologies and services the students performed in the agency or in the homes. Assessments were conducted to determine the need for the teaching or the services. Interestingly, the agency staff benefited a great deal from the teaching sessions. They listened attentively to the mini-teaching presentations that lasted from 1 to 5 minutes and to the lengthier major teaching presentations. The students learned from each other and freely admitted that some of the information shared was new to them. I found myself advising the students that they should shorten their presentations when giving them to the elderly clients. Eventually, the students found greater success in evaluating their clients' learning when shorter sessions were held with less information shared.

Our entire clinical group participated in the health fair held on the GMU campus during the semester. We conducted blood pressure and vision screenings. This experience provided an opportunity to interact with adult clients across a wide range of ages. Health fair participants were grateful for the screenings offered and listened intently to the student teaching about healthy behaviors to control blood pressure. Some were surprised about their inability to read the Snellen eye chart to their satisfaction. I supervised the students and offered active assistance when they were busy in the booths. I allowed the students multiple opportunities to teach clients after I modeled the behavior at the beginning of the day. We developed sheets that were used to report our findings. We were careful to add a disclaimer that our findings were a gross assessment at best and were not to be construed as definitive findings. Those visitors with questionable findings were referred to their health-care providers.

Specific topics that were presented to the participants, residents, and families at the senior center included:

- Sources of fats in foods—Benefit or risk?
- Estrogen and osteoporosis
- What it means to be the caregiver of an elderly person
- Sources of calcium and how much we need to stay healthy
- Choosing and proper care of hearing aids
- Safe handling and administration of medicines
- Orthostatic hypotension

This teaching and learning strategy was very effective in achieving the goal of imparting information to the clients and their families, but it also provided a valuable means of learning for the students.

Preconferences and postconferences were important to the students and to me. In preconference, we discussed each student's objectives and the plan for the day to achieve those objectives. This seemed to be comforting to the students and a way to ease into the clinical day. It also afforded them an opportunity to ask me questions to clarify assignments. The co-director would be given the opportunity to make announcements or share information about the current participants or new participants. We collaborated with the nurse in the adult day-care center and the nurse in the assisted living area regarding client status and medication administration. If someone was in need of a home visit, we were informed and planned how this would be accomplished.

Some clients were suspected of having reactions to medications, and our students were assigned home visits to monitor them. Keep in mind that the home visits for the assisted living clients were conducted in the clients' apartments on-site. Students achieved a renewed appreciation for the varied definitions of home, family, and community.

The first class to be assigned to this community-based site, the senior center, was energetic and enthusiastic. Although it took all of us some time to determine our unique roles, we were committed to a positive experience for the clients, agency, and students. The students collaborated with all interested parties to keep the clients as the first priority and to help them maintain their health and prevent illness. Although we were not able to halt the aging process, we were successful in achieving a great deal of learning for everyone.

References

Andresen, EM, et al. (1998). Selecting a generic measure of health-related quality of life for use among older adults. A comparison of candidate instruments. Eval Health Prof 21(2), 244–264.

Kandzari, JH, & Howard, JR (1981). Family health protective behaviors assessment tool. In: The well family: A developmental approach to assessment. Boston: Little, Brown, & Co.

Rowe, JW, & Kahn, RL (1999). Six myths about aging: Getting up in years doesn't mean you're getting down in your ability to thrive. The Washington Post 15(29), 12.

Wissmann, JL, & Wilmoth, MC (1996). Meeting the learning needs of senior citizens and nursing students through a community-based pharmacology experience. J Community Health Nurs 13(3), 159–165.

Yoder, MH, et al. (1997). Agency-university collaboration: Home care early in the student curriculum. Home Health Nurse 15(7), 493–499.

CHAPTER 8

Teaching Students the Care of Underserved Children in an Elementary School

Carol J. Heddleston

Learning Objectives

1) Describe the faculty role in developing an elementary school as a site for community-based practice.
2) List effective communication techniques that can be used in this setting.
3) Define students' scope of nursing practice.
4) Describe effective learning experiences and teaching strategies to assist students to use their previously acquired knowledge and skills in the elementary school setting.
5) Enhance critical-thinking and therapeutic-intervention skills, through students' work in an elementary school setting.

Health care is among the most complex of services to deliver cooperatively. Collaboration between local education agencies and a university-based school of nursing can result in a wide range of benefits to pre-kindergarten to 12th grade students and their families. These are in addition to the benefits to graduate and undergraduate nursing students, the faculties of both the university and the agencies, and the community at large. Yet, there are relatively few effective and long-lasting models of such collaboration, and there are barriers to initial and long-range success.

Agency personnel are seeking health-care services for their students, sometimes for the families of their students, or for the community at large. The university faculty is seeking training opportunities for their students, faculty practice sites, and research opportunities. One can envision the two groups facing each other and reaching out to connect. (DeLellis1998).

GENERAL CONCEPTS FOR FACULTY IN AN ELEMENTARY SCHOOL SETTING

As a faculty member using an elementary school as a community-based site, you must have certain knowledge, skills, and attitudes to be a successful teacher. First, you must be familiar with the school itself. Although you can become familiar in a variety of ways, a visit and tour of the school is usually the best. Meeting with the principal, the vice-principal, and the school nurse is helpful in the early planning stages. During this meeting it's important to clarify the expectations of school personnel regarding the student placement. You must also have knowledge of the community resources available, and visiting the public health department can be of great help.

A windshield tour of the surrounding community is a good way to see the community from a child's or family's point of view. It is a good idea to become familiar with the shopping facilities, closest hospital, churches, recreational facilities, libraries, and so forth. Also investigate the availability of public transportation. Safety is another issue to evaluate. Is the neighborhood safe for children and older adults to walk in? Will student nurses be safe visiting students' families in this neighborhood? Plan to spend at least 2 days getting familiar with the school and the surrounding community.

The number one skill you will need to be a successful faculty member in the school setting is the ability to effectively communicate. The ability to listen is invaluable, as are good verbal, nonverbal, and writing skills. All of the previous interpersonal skills you have used successfully in the past will be needed here. Develop a good working relationship with the principal and the teaching staff and, most important, with your students. I discovered, with students especially, it is best to put things in writing. They have a lot to remember and can refer to written information later (Table 8–1). It is also helpful to write a weekly newsletter that can be distributed to teachers' mailboxes, informing them about the students' capabilities and what they will be doing weekly to meet course objectives (Table 8–2).

Other skills needed to be a successful faculty member in this setting are the abilities to work independently, that is, to be self-directed, and to help students be self-directed. Strong critical-thinking skills are also essential, so that you are able to make sound decisions and use good judgment when difficult situations arise. One example of a situation that often arises is the teachers not understanding the role of the student nurse in the classroom. Many of them see the student as an extra pair of hands and try to use them like teacher's aides. Situations such as these, if they occur often, will defeat the purpose of the program. Encourage your students to handle such problems by themselves, if at all possible. Often, the students bring the problems they are encountering to the postconference meeting, and the group as a whole will offer solutions. This is an excellent way for students to develop critical-thinking skills.

The ability to be flexible is another desirable behavior to cultivate. Each day in the school setting, new, unpredictable situations and challenges arise. The teachers often reschedule planned teaching sessions, there are snow days and sick days, and the regular teacher may not be in school the day you and your students need him or her to be there. The scheduling of home visits is the one activity that requires the most flexibility. Many times families will not be home even though the nursing student has called in advance. Sometimes the family will just not answer the door or will send someone else to answer and say they are not there. So, always have a Plan B.

As a faculty member in a community-based setting, you not only have to be knowledgeable about the school environment, the student population served, and the community surrounding it, you also must be able to communicate with all the people you deal with each day. In these dealings, a positive attitude is extremely important. You must be aware that your students are looking to you for guidance and instructions. Be a role model for them, demonstrating professional behavior at all times, including maintaining a professional appearance, being trustworthy, and maintaining confidentiality.

You teach to learn yourself, and there is always more to learn, especially when dealing with the unique differences in the people you encounter.

FACULTY APPLICATIONS IN COMMUNITY-BASED SITES

Developing The Site

H Elementary School is a science and math focus school located in Fairfax County, Virginia. The facility has a student population of approximately 500 children in grades kindergarten through 6th grade. Students attending the school come from a variety of socioeconomic backgrounds. The breakdown of the population is as follows: American Indian/Alaskan: 0.4 percent; Hispanic: 10.1 percent; African-American: 48.6 percent; Caucasian: 27.6 percent; other: 13.3 percent. Forty-six

Table 8-1

Initial Orientation Letter for Nursing Students

Dear Nursing 341 Students:

This is my third time teaching this course at School. I think it went very well the first two times, and I am hoping for an even better semester this year. There are a few things I feel are important to share with you at the start.

I hope we can have open lines of communication at all times. Please do not hesitate to call me at home or on my cell phone at any time. I do want you to e-mail me your journals each week by Monday at noon for the previous week. In your journals feel free to tell me your thoughts and feelings. Also, to help me at the end in your evaluations and to keep you focused, tell me what objectives you met that week. Please understand I will keep these journals confidential and share them only after asking your permission.

This semester I will be doing something new to keep the teachers and staff informed. This is writing a weekly newsletter about what we are doing there. I will need your help with this, but I think we will all benefit from it, because the teachers will know where you should be in your coursework and also what you are accomplishing on a weekly basis.

For the first few days you will be learning the "ropes." As soon as possible, you will need to give a schedule of when you will and will not be in the classroom to the teacher you will be assigned to and keep it accurate and up to date. This schedule should be for a month at a time, and the forms for this have been provided for you. As you will see, you must keep your teacher informed, or things will not go well for you. Your teacher trusts that you will be there when you say you will.

We will be having daily preconferences and postconferences in the space assigned to us at 0745 and 1330. You need to put in 6 hours of work each day for 28 days. This time will be logged in on your clinical time sheet. You should probably bring lunch or plan to eat with the children in the cafeteria. If there are school closings, you need to plan to do productive work on your projects; we may meet at GMU during the Fairfax County School Spring Break. If you can think of something that you would like the group to do during this time, let me know.

You will be making home visits in pairs and you will learn more about this from the Fairfax County Health Department. Our health-promotion, disease-prevention focus will be on ASTHMA. You will learn a lot about asthma, and I expect most of your health teaching to revolve around asthma. You will have a special orientation to the ASTHMA PROJECT soon. Early on, try to find a child in your classroom who has asthma. Try to follow him or her for the semester and make arrangements to visit the family. You need to plan on making at least two home visits for each case.

The projects that you will do will require that you network, get resources and supplies, and do some research. You will need to find out what health education is needed from the teacher and also from your observations in the classroom. For instance, if you are teaching dental hygiene, you will need to get toothbrushes and paste for the children from the dental society or a dentist you know. You can also get information and handouts from a variety of sources but you must be creative and resourceful. One of the topics we are always asked to teach is HAND WASHING, because this is a big health issue at this time. I have some ideas about how this was done before, and the children loved it.

When you are doing a teaching project, you should observe how the teacher presents new material and what teaching methods are effective for your particular age group. Try to capitalize on the teacher's knowledge and expertise. We have the READY-SET-GO health curriculum available to us, and you can certainly use its ideas for your projects. Remember when doing these teaching projects to use the steps in the nursing process (assessment, planning, implementation, and evaluation).

You may be involved in some health screenings, such as vision and hearing, and also may do some head checks for lice. This is done when you are assigned to the health clinic aide or at his or her request. We will only be observing in the health room, and you will not give medications in this setting.

I think you will find me fairly reasonable when it comes to turning in assignments; but you will be downgraded if you habitually turn things in late and tend to take advantage of my kindness! This course has only three process recordings, a teaching plan, and a family assessment as written assignments, so I feel that should not be a burden on anyone.

Professionalism is one of the things that I value the most when it comes to evaluating you in this course. We will discuss this a lot more, but I feel that this is an area where you can really shine in the setting we are in. This means when you tell someone that you will do something or be somewhere that you will do it and can be counted on and trusted to follow through.

You will have a lot of free time to use in various ways, and you must be creative and show initiative with your teaching projects or whatever you decide to do.

Most of all let's have a lot of fun, learn a lot, and build on what we already know. I am really looking forward to watching you grow!

Sincerely,

Carol Heddleston, RN, MN

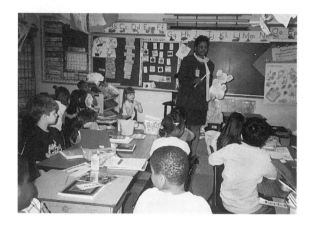

Table 8-2
GMU Student Nurses Notes

Dear Teachers and Staff:

We had a very productive week this past week. We were able to identify most of the students who have already been diagnosed with asthma. We are hoping to start making home visits soon on all of the kindergarten and first grade students that have been identified.

We also were able to do at least one health promotion lesson in each class, and I believe the students did a good job. This was the first experience in teaching children for most of the group. Any feedback you can give them is always appreciated.

Thank you for allowing the student nurses to practice their skills in doing health promotion and disease prevention in the school setting. Please do not forget our blood pressure screenings each Tuesday AM in the teachers lounge.

Carol J. Heddleston, GMU Clinical Instructor

---

percent of the students receive free or reduced-price lunch. Because there are many children who are military dependents or come from single-parent families, the mobility rate is about 30 percent of the students per year.

The staff for the school includes the principal, assistant principal, a media specialist, and a clinic aide, in addition to four secretaries who do the administrative work. The Fairfax County Public Health Department provides the school nurse. A social worker and a counselor also work in the school. There are about 25 teachers in the classroom setting and several resource teachers. There is a gifted and talented program, a learning disabilities program, a Title I and reading resource program, and an English-as-a-second-language program. Because H Elementary is a science and math focus school, there is a science and a math resource teacher. Also, the school participates in a technology program that provides students and staff with Internet capability throughout the facility.

Four other schools share Fairfax County's school health nurse. As a result, she is only at the school on a very part-time basis, and her main role is to be a health resource and to do consultation. She is responsible for the supervision and training of the clinic room aide and acts as a liaison between students, staff, family, and community. The school health nurse also is a case manager and multidisciplinary team member. She participates in any child abuse and neglect investigations and will do home and classroom assessments when asked. The clinic room aide has the main responsibility of caring for sick and injured children. She also does all of the vision and hearing screening, assists with giving medications and tracking immunizations, and refers any students with health needs to the school health nurse.

The initial contact for the use of this elementary school as a community-based site was made through the college's clinical site coordinator. Box 8–1 can be used by faculty to orient themselves to school settings. Another elementary school in the county had piloted this program and received a good response, thus paving the way for another school to agree to allow student nurses to use the site. The Fairfax County Public Health Department nursing education research coordinator was the key person for making policies for the student nurses to follow while in the school setting. Several meetings between the principal, the nursing instructor, and the school health nurse were conducted before the student nurses arrived. The first meeting was conducted to discuss roles and responsibilities, student assignments, and activities for the semester. This helped with creating a good working relationship between all concerned and with allowing each person to voice concerns and goals

> **Box 8-1** Learning Exercise for Faculty Use
>
> ## Faculty Orientation
>
> Use the following questions to begin your orientation as a faculty member assigned to a school setting:
>
> What is the size and demographics of the populations of the school?
>
> Who are the administrative, support, and teaching staff of the school?
>
> What types of programs does the school offer?
>
> Is there a school nurse on-site? Is the nurse part of the school staff or part of a local health department?
>
> Does the school have a specific health curriculum?
>
> What kind of meetings or written forms of communication may be used to orient the teachers and others to the student's role and function within the school?

for the program. Students were oriented to School Health Services by the Fairfax County Public Health Department before entering the school setting. This orientation was a comprehensive introduction to school health nursing.

The Fairfax County Public Health Department was responsible for arranging any experiences in school or health department sites other than the assigned school. There were several field trips to other types of community-based settings, such as The K Center, which is a school that provides services for students with severe disabilities and moderate retardation. A trip to an agency that deals with speech and hearing loss in children was also made available.

The nursing students were typically assigned to a classroom teacher to facilitate the coordination of teaching projects and access to a family within that classroom setting. The principal was very open to allowing the student nurses into the classroom to conduct health-promotion and disease-prevention teaching projects. Health curriculum existed for each grade level in the elementary school. A manual, called *Ready, Set, Go for Good Health* (1991), contained certain topics with predeveloped teaching plans that could be presented. Unfortunately, teachers in the school rarely had the time or the inclination to follow this curriculum. Thus, there was a wonderful opportunity for student nurses to find their niche in this setting.

To meet course objectives, the student nurses needed to make home visits. The school health nurse did not have the time to make these type of visits, although she would have liked to do so. The principal of the school asked that we select a student that the teacher suggested could benefit from a visit, and then the principal called the family and told them the purpose of the visit. This method seemed to work well in all but a few cases.

Effective Communication Strategies

From the beginning of the relationship between the College of Nursing and the H Elementary School, the most important need was that of effective communication. There was much new territory being explored and many different people being affected by the presence of student nurses in this setting. Everyone needed to know that we were going to be at the school for the next 14 weeks. The elementary school had a staff newsletter that was printed weekly and distributed to all teachers and staff, including cafeteria workers, janitors, and anyone else in the building. This was the main form of written communication we used to tell everyone about the student nurses working at the school. All of the teachers were asked if they would like to have a student nurse in their classrooms, and that was how it was decided where each student would be based. The student nurses were allowed to choose which grade level they would prefer, and, for the most part, most of them were happy with their assignment.

The first day that the student nurses were in the school happened to be a teacher workday, and the children were not present. This was a perfect opportunity for student nurses and teachers to meet and get some kind of a relationship started. Each student nurse accompanied his or her teacher to the classroom to get an idea of the physical layout and also to be given the *Ready, Set, Go for Good Health* manual. At this time the student nurses were told to tell the teachers what the objectives for the clinical experience would be. I believe the student nurses were not effective in communicating clearly about the objectives at that time, because, as the semester progressed, there were always questions about what the students were supposed to be doing. The principal preferred a very loose arrangement, because she felt that when things came up, the student could seize whatever opportunity was presented. This worked well in some situations, but not in all classes. Many teachers were comfortable with "going with the flow," and others were not. The main problem was that the teachers saw student nurses as student teachers. They could identify with this idea, because they themselves had been student teachers, and they knew what the expectations were for this role. Teachers wanted the student nurses in the classroom the whole day, and they did not understand when the nurse was only present for a short period and had to leave to pursue some other task. I learned that the instructor must be able to step in at this point to clarify the role of the student and try to alleviate some of the misunderstanding. The student nurses were not able to do this effectively. About halfway through the semester, a second meeting was called so that any problems could be discussed and the role of the student nurses clarified.

Looking back, I can see where a weekly newsletter about what the goals for that particular week were could have been most useful. I am now doing this and including it in the staff weekly paper, and this seems to have made a world of difference in defining what the student nurses are supposed to be doing.

Guidelines for Supervision of Students

Each clinical group is made up of many personalities, ages, and cultural backgrounds, and therefore, it is difficult to clearly state what level of supervision may be needed in the school setting. For the most part, the older, more mature student seems to "take off" in the elementary school setting. At first, students were given some guidelines, but soon they were totally autonomous. The students who had backgrounds in another field seemed to feel totally at ease when given few constraints on their initiatives. The younger students, however, seemed to want and demand more supervision. They wanted constant guidance on what they should be doing and when. They were not as skilled in interpersonal relationship building, and they wanted the instructor to tell them how to initiate contact with families. It is part of the learning process. One of the teaching strategies that seemed to help students with interpersonal relations was to role-play during the postconference time. They would be given a scenario and would then practice what to say using therapeutic communication techniques. They seemed to like these practice sessions.

In the area of making a home visit, much guidance and supervision was needed as well. These students had never done anything like this before, and they were very unskilled in dealing with situations that were unstructured. Students needed to relate with not only children and their teachers, but also with parents and disciplines such as social services and speech therapists. They were doing these things very early in their nursing school careers. This ability to deal with other disciplines is of great value in their future roles, as noted by Passarelli: "The evolving role of the school nurse includes a shift of health-care delivery to the community setting. The efficacy and access of community-based care delivery will require nurses to have greater program development and management skills. It will also ... highlight the need to hone interdisciplinary and intradisciplinary teamwork skills" (1994, p 141).

One of the areas the student nurses seemed to particularly enjoy was working in the school health clinic. However, it was felt that this was not a good setting for the students to practice their skills because of the constraints placed on them by the state. The clinic room aide must follow very strict guidelines when dealing with illness or injury in the school setting. She is not allowed to make a diagnosis or give treatment, other than apply ice or give a Band-Aid. She must call a parent or guardian to pick up

Chapter 8 | *Teaching Students the Care of Underserved Children in an Elementary School*

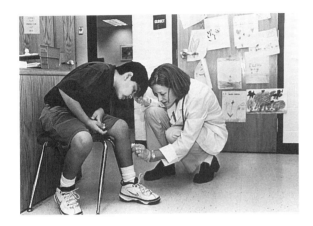

a child with a certain degree of fever or a child who is vomiting. Therefore, according to a memorandum from the Fairfax County Public Health Department's Nursing Research Coordinator, "Student nurses may observe in the clinic to gain an understanding of the role of the clinic room aide, but this should not be the focus for either the junior or senior level student. Because the student nurses have not completed the 35-hour orientation for providing care to sick and injured students, the student nurse may *not* under any circumstances cover the clinic in the absence of the clinic room aide."

DEFINITION OF SCOPE OF NURSING PRACTICE

This course gave the student an opportunity to provide collaborative nursing care to a population of children who were culturally diverse and vulnerable. The main focus was health promotion and disease prevention for students, families, and small groups. There was also an emphasis on refining therapeutic communication skills that could be easily practiced each day.

Some of the activities that students were involved in to practice their nursing skills included developing a health education project, performing a health and wellness assessment, doing vision and hearing screening on new students to the school, conducting a home visit for assessment of health education needs, performing nutrition assessments and counseling, assessing growth and development, and planning and implementing a health fair at the school.

Very early in the semester, the student nurses were encouraged to develop a simple health education project to present to their individual classes or the entire grade, if possible. They felt comfortable teaching about hand washing because that was the first clinical skill they had been taught in clinical lab. In addition, the school principal voiced the great need for this topic to be reinforced often because of the prevalence of the cold and flu virus in the school setting. Every grade level was taught how to wash hands correctly, why it is so important, and when it should be done. In some of the 4th, 5th, and 6th grade classes, the nurses used a black light and "germ" dust to show how easily germs were spread by way of dirty hands. The students really enjoyed this type of presentation. As an additional reminder to students, posters about germs were posted in each bathroom throughout the school.

Dental hygiene was another popular topic chosen by the student nurses to teach in the various grade levels. Because February is dental health month, the timing of this project was perfect. The student nurses first had to make phone calls and then visit the Northern Virginia Dental Association. They were able to borrow the Association's puppet and a large toothbrush for demonstrating proper brushing technique. They were also provided with a video on good dental habits that the younger age groups seemed to really enjoy. All of the student nurses had to come up with sources for free toothbrushes, and some were even able to obtain entire kits that had the paste and the plaque-detecting tablets in them. The project allowed the student nurses to begin to understand about how to access community resources.

Nutrition was the third topic that all of the student nurses taught to the various age groups. Most of them ate lunch with their class once or twice during the semester, and during this time they were able to assess what was served at lunch and how much of it the children actually ate. The kindergarten students brought a snack each day because they did not go to the cafeteria when on half-day schedules. The student nurses were easily able to make a nursing diagnosis of poor nutritional intake due to lack of knowledge of food groups. Again, many resources were used to present classes that had good content about food groups, and the student nurses were able to provide "healthy snack feasts" in almost every class they taught. They had to access many community resources to make these a success. They were able to get handouts from the American Dairy Association, the American Heart Association, and the American Cancer Society, in addition to some food donations from a grocery store. In a few cases, they brought the food in at their own expense.

It was during the time that the student nurses were developing their own teaching skills that they also realized that they were developing other skills, such as assessing growth and development, fine and gross motor skills, and socialization and cognitive skills of the children in their classes. With the teacher's guidance they were able to choose the child that might benefit from a home visit and a family assessment. They then were allowed to look at the child's school record to learn a little more about his or her background and previous history, both medical and social.

The principal was the first person to ask the child's family if a student nurse could come for a home visit. Usually, the family would say that it would be fine for us to come. However, scheduling an appointment was not always easy and was a time when the student nurses' communication skills were greatly challenged. The nursing students needed to be assertive but sensitive to the fact that they were going to be entering another person's private space. Many of the student nurses felt very uncomfortable at first about going into a home of a child from the school.

EFFECTIVE LEARNING EXPERIENCES AND TEACHING STRATEGIES USED

As can be determined after reading this chapter, the use of the elementary school as a community-based site for the practice of nursing offered many great opportunities for student learning. The student nurses learned how to develop and teach a lesson plan to a group of elementary students. They also learned how to access community resources, develop therapeutic relationships with children and their families, make a home visit and do a family assessment, and plan and implement a health fair for the school community.

The teaching strategies included such things as role-playing and trying out techniques on each other before trying them on families. The students watched a faculty member enact what might happen in a home visit situation and were allowed to practice on each other first. To lessen the anxiety of being totally alone and responsible for what might happen, two students would go together with the instructor on the first visit. One student was to be the eyes and ears and was not to talk, and the other student was to focus on the family member or members and practice therapeutic communication skills. Students had already been exposed to writing process recordings, so they had a fairly extensive knowledge about what therapeutic communication techniques to use and what types of communication were not considered therapeutic. The school health nurse told students about the necessity of bringing some type of pamphlet or other handout about topics that may be of interest when going on these visits. The students therefore had to do a lot of preparation in advance and be ready with answers about health questions that a family member might have. Again, this provided the nursing student with another opportunity to access community resources.

One of the children visited by the students had Crohn's disease and had recently had surgery for the purpose of creating a temporary colostomy. The student nurse obtained information from the local Ostomy Association and brought handouts from them to the first visit. We also visited a child with diabetes, and the student nurse was able to bring the family a lot of information from the Juvenile Diabetes Association and to tell them about a camp that was for children with diabetes. Students were instructed that, when faced with a question for which they had no answer, they should say they did not know but would find out and get back to the family with the information they needed. This was a good way for the student nurse to be able to go back for a follow-up visit.

Students were given a format for the family assessment, and they had the questions they needed to ask in advance. But it was not easy to get all of the information during one visit. The students were told to find out as much as possible about the family before the visit. Such preparation helped to lower some of the stress of not knowing what to expect. Nursing students had to collaborate with the school health nurse to see if she knew anything about the child or his or her family. They also collaborated with

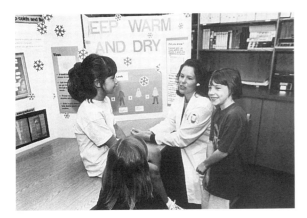

 Chapter 8 | *Teaching Students the Care of Underserved Children in an Elementary School*

the school social worker and the school counselor in some situations. These professionals had already spoken to the parents and could give the student valuable information. The school principal seemed to be the best source of knowledge about a students' family situations, and the nursing students soon learned to collaborate with her often. The school also had a parent resource person who spoke Spanish, and she went with them on a visit where the family spoke only Spanish.

The final project for nursing students to plan and implement was the community health fair. This project allowed them to put all of their teaching skills and abilities to practice in a few short, but intense, hours. Best of all, they brought together all of the resources they had found over the semester and used pamphlets and teaching aides, such as breast and testicular models, to teach the community about health promotion and disease prevention. They were able to do blood pressure and diabetes screenings, and they even had a stress-reduction booth.

The target population for the health fair was the teachers and staff of the school as well as parents and the surrounding community. The students had to develop ways to inform all of these people about the fair, and this further challenged their communication skills. They had to write an article for the parents' newsletter and the local newspaper. They also made posters and flyers to distribute in the neighborhood. The health fair was an excellent way for a community-based clinical in an elementary school to end the semester.

How to Use Exemplars of Student Narratives to Enhance Learning Experiences

Perhaps the best source of student narratives was the journals they wrote each week to tell the instructor their thoughts and feeling and also to give examples of how they met the course objectives. A journal is an excellent tool for evaluating the critical-thinking skills throughout the clinical course (Callister 1993). It is especially valuable in this type of clinical experience because the instructor is not able to be present during all of the students' interactions with clients.

The nursing students are able to gain insight into their behavior and, as a result, are usually aware of what they did well and where improvements can be made. The instructor can also give feedback on a weekly basis and can give ideas for areas that need more work. I required my students to e-mail me their previous week's journals before we met again. This allowed me to give them immediate feedback and was not terribly time consuming.

Some students' critical-thinking and communication skills were more fully developed than others. One particular student was not only gifted in these areas, but was also very enthusiastic and quite verbal about what she learned and how she applied her knowledge.

 Tuesday, 02/17/98: I woke up this morning knowing that this is going to be a busy day. I have two presentations of the Heart Teaching Project (different first grade classes), and in between I have my first home visit. Needless to say, I am so excited and a little anxious thinking about my clinical today....

When I got to my clinical site, there was nothing out of the ordinary. My partner (Kara) and I got together just to make sure that we didn't forget any of our materials. Then, our preconference started. After the conference, I made my call to the family I am visiting. The father answered the phone, and I could have sworn that my heart skipped a beat. To my surprise, he didn't give me any hassle and he nicely gave the phone to his wife. Talking to Ms. B was quite reassuring. I felt that she really wants to meet with us and perhaps we will even be able to assess what help we can offer her. Once I replaced the receiver on the phone, I began my walk to my first task of the day—the first teaching project presentation....

The teaching went extremely well, and I didn't feel nervous at all because I already know these children, their abilities, and their limitations (after observing them in the classroom during the time that I am in clinical—this is part of my assessment for the teaching plan). Kara did very well in her part too, and with teamwork we managed to keep the attention of 15 5-6 year-olds, for a little over an hour and a half, teaching them about the heart, nutrition, and exercise....

Immediately after the teaching, I met with Carol (my instructor) and Jennifer (my fellow nursing student) to discuss our approach for our home visit. Then, off we went to the client's home, with my heart pounding and my mind racing....

Even though different individuals have told me about the living conditions of the family that I was about to visit, I still wasn't sure what to expect. I decided that for myself, the best thing to do is to erase any preconceived notions (on my part) and any past input from others. In this way I can start with a clean slate, whereby everything that I write and observe will be my own, when I am actually at the site.

The first view of the muddy and basically messed up yard (in the pouring rain) gave me my first impression of the low SES of this family, thus enabling me to keep an objective mind when I went into the actual house and met some of the family members. Thus I would assess the family without the idea that they are just lazy or unhygienic; rather it is the poor access to resources that I should focus on.

Meeting Ms. B was such an eye-opener. I was expecting a young, clueless mother of five who was both bashful and defensive. Yet, I met an intelligent (quite informed) young woman, who almost had an air of confidence in her, or at least that's the image that she projected to us.

Her concerns and knowledge about some health issues regarding her son astonished me. And I found her quite open and receptive. After discussing various aspects of what our (nursing students') tasks are and what we can offer as help to her, we bid goodbye, with hope that we would be able to visit again and make a difference in my client's (my student's) life, if not his family's. I practiced observing and gathering data by simply watching and listening. And I found myself making mental assessments during and after the interview. I found this visit quite refreshing. I started out this semester not knowing what assessment, care plan, and resource project I can do for the different courses that I have this semester. It looks like I can do all the projects with just using one client as a focus.

When I got back from the visit, Kara and I presented our teaching project to her class. This went very well too, even though I found myself a little nervous as I ventured into new and unknown territory.

Overall, this day has been quite exhausting but definitely interesting. I learned a lot today—from technical and practical (gathering data, interpersonal communication, assessment, teaching) to character building (adapting, flexibility, and going with the flow of events, collaborating and interacting with people of various ages and status).

Thursday, 02/19/98: I expected today to be one of a relaxed nature compared to last Tuesday. I didn't have anything planned particularly today, except to research both my oral hygiene presentation for next week, and find facts and resources about obesity and diabetes mellitus. Luckily, I had a surprise for the day—we got to visit Harriet (PHN) at the health department. Even though the building itself was nothing from the ordinary, it was certainly refreshing to find so many resources and pamphlets that I can use for my clinical. I was quite disappointed though that it seems the Health Dept. has such a limited health-promotion focus (prenatal, STDs and immunizations). But I did get some ideas for further teaching, such as lead poisoning. While we were there, Harriet got a phone call regarding pin worms, so we got to discuss and talk about this parasite, which helped me review what I already know about it (from my Med Tech years).

When we got back to the school, one of my classmates was having trouble with her assigned teacher. It is through this that I realized that not everyone has the same clinical experience. I am having the time of my life, keeping myself organized, basically doing things that I want to do (related to health promotion), and managing my own time. All of this was possible because I communicated to my teacher from the beginning what I was there to do and what my plan was. I was also blessed with such an open-minded and kind and cooperative teacher.

In the following journal entry, it is clear that another student was lacking confidence before the home visit, but he prepared himself well. He planned what he was going to discuss with the family about food allergies and researched some community resources before the visit. In addition, he was able to give them some pamphlets about the problem the student was having. His preparation helped him feel more relaxed, and the visit was a success.

04/13/99 I arrived at the clinical site at 8.00am for final preparation on my home visit scheduled at 9.00am. I was concerned about what to expect from my clients whom I understood had basic knowledge about medications. I was also concerned about not giving them the impression that I was an amateur, or incompetent.

My objective was based on how to overcome these concerns and have them develop trust and confidence in me. I think I was able to accomplish my objectives, as I was able to offer them some helpful hints about food allergy and answered some of the questions they had. I particularly believe the pamphlets I gave them will be a good source of additional information they may have regarding the food allergy.

I proposed rescheduling for a follow-up to furnish the family with some information they had requested, which I couldn't provide an immediate answer at the time of the visit.

It was a positive experience for me.

Another goal for students to achieve in this community-based setting is cultural competence. One of the licensed practical nurses in this course was very interested in diabetes education. She was able to visit a family of a child who had this disorder and do some teaching about its medical management. The added challenge was that the mother only spoke Spanish, so the student asked the Spanish-speaking parent liaison coordinator from the school to accompany her on this visit. It was extremely important that the student recognized ways to become culturally competent: the problem was a topic for a pre-conference meeting before her visit.

4/30/99 Last week was my family health assessment with A.'s family. I wish we could have done the assessment with A. there, I really feel like only 50% of the assessment was done since she wasn't really included. I have met her briefly before to do her hearing/visual screening exam, but of course that didn't focus on her diabetes at all.

After talking with her mother I feel like they have a fairly good handle on things and are feeling more comfortable with her diagnosis. Her mother seemed at ease with the insulin and administration of it, although she wasn't aware of the need to rotate sites and the purpose of that. She also had some concerns about when A. is sick and how to go about taking her insulin and how much. I basically informed her that it's important for her to always take the insulin and to eat as well to avoid a hypoglycemic reaction ... suggested small frequent meals, food that's light on the stomach, and to contact her doctor's office because she might benefit more from a sliding scale coverage plan.

I also tried to stress the importance of having some glucotabs or something similar at school in case of an emergency. Also a medic alert bracelet should be obtained ASAP. I also tried to express the need to get all the family members of the house involved and especially to know the signs/symptoms of hypo/hyperglycemia since they are around a lot of the time as well. I'm glad I got to go on this home visit rather than the one that concerned the ADHD child just because I do have a special interest in diabetes and especially secondary care for it. I am looking into becoming a certified diabetic educator. Muchas gracias!

For students in the community-based setting of an elementary school that enrolls underserved children to become sensitive to other cultures, they must first become aware of their own cultural heritage. This group of student nurses was itself very culturally diverse, so the students themselves often addressed these issues. Students also must be aware of the client's culture as described by the client. Often it is easy to stereotype people, and it is important to listen to the clients' descriptions of their cultural beliefs and practices. Likewise, a student must be aware of the adaptations clients make to live in North America. Children adapt quickly, but parents are much slower to make changes. Finally, the student must formulate the nursing care plan to incorporate the culture of the client. This is particularly important in a case such as the previously mentioned Hispanic child with diabetes mellitus (Kittler & Sucher 1994).

It is easily understood how many issues nursing students in this school setting address in one short semester. Critical-thinking skills are developed on a daily basis. Therapeutic communication techniques are practiced and enhanced. Previously acquired knowledge and skills are applied in several new situations. There was a tremendous amount of growth in the students' self-confidence after they did all of the teaching projects, the home visits, and the family assessments. The health fair they planned and implemented was the final proof that they could teach health-promotion and disease-prevention strategies to individuals and small groups in a variety of settings.

According to Pierce and Mitchell, "...health-care delivery continues to shift away from the hospital-centered, inpatient treatment to community sites such as outpatient centers, churches, homes, public schools, and the workplace. Nurses may find increasing employment outside of hospitals as all types of existing and newly developed health-care systems seek qualified nurses. These changes will continue to boost the demand for case managers and those with 'independent clinical decision-making skills'" (2000 p 17). The health system will focus on entire populations and nurses will provide effective programs for health promotion and disease prevention, identifying risk factors and detecting illness in its early stages (Pierce & Mitchell 2000). It is with this trend in mind that students in the community-based elementary school setting are being prepared to meet the health-care needs of the future.

References

Callister, LC (1993). The use of student journal in nursing education: Making meaning out of clinical experiences. J Nurs Educ 32,185–186.

DeLellis, AJ (1998). Collaboration between school of nursing and local education agencies to provide health care services to pre-kindergarten through twelfth grade students: Elements of cooperative agreements. Pub Health Nurs 15(2), 104–108.

Kittler, PG, & Sucher, KP (1994). Diet counseling in a multicultural society. Diabetes Educ 16(2), 127–134.

Passereli, C (1994). School Nursing: Trends for the Future. J Sch Health 64(4), 141–143.

Pierce, C, & Mitchell, P (2000). Picture yourself in nursing's active market. Nursing 2000 Career Directory, 17–18.

Ready, Set, Go for Good Health (1991). Elementary Health Education. Fairfax County Public Schools. Fairfax, VA.

CHAPTER 9

Teaching Students in a Campus Clinical

M. Lucille Boland

Learning Objectives

1) Identify the preliminary organizational work that needs to occur prior to the beginning of the clinical course.

2) Develop several appropriate student projects prior to the beginning of the clinical course.

3) Discuss student expectations with regard to the community-based clinical course.

4) Develop a rotation schedule for the students during the clinical experience.

5) Identify a plan for evaluation of the clinical placement units.

6) Explore methods of student evaluation in an unstructured clinical setting.

After the decision has been made to develop a community-based curriculum, the next logical step is to identify clinical sites that will allow students to develop the skills necessary to function in a multidisciplinary health-focused arena. A college campus is a fertile site for instituting such a student clinical experience in a community-based curriculum. The literature is replete with studies of health issues that focus on the college student and on nursing's involvement with these issues. Consider the major health issues on a college campus: alcohol and substance abuse, eating disorders, depression and suicide, high-risk sexual behavior, and sexually transmitted diseases, to name a few. Each issue has a substantial amount of research or emphasis in the literature. For example, on the issue of alcohol and substance abuse, Conyne and colleagues (1994), Haspel (1998), McNair and colleagues (1998), Miller (1997), and Wall and coworkers (1998) all deal with various aspects of alcohol or substance abuse from outcome expectancies and attitudes toward drinking to the use of primary prevention precepts in setting up programs on campuses. In the area of eating disorders, Georgiou and colleagues (1997), Heatherton and coworkers (1995), Mangweth and coworkers (1995), and Seymour and colleagues (1997) focus on the instances of eating disorders, lifestyle practices, and eating habits of college-aged students. Depression and suicide was addressed by Roehrig and Range (1995) when they looked at predicting suicidality in college students. Last, high-risk sexual behavior and sexually transmitted diseases have voluminous citations in the literature, including that of Ho and colleagues (1998),

Maticka-Tyndale and colleagues (1998), Minoia (1996), Prince and coworkers (1998), and American Health Consultants Inc. (1994), who focused on sexual behavior as well as specific sexually transmitted diseases such as HIV and human papillomavirus. The college campus of today provides ample opportunities for nursing students to learn the role of a community-based nurse as well as to have an impact on the health of a vulnerable population.

The question then becomes, how does one go about developing a viable, meaningful clinical for students in such a community-based curriculum? Following is a discussion of how one professor approached the task for the first time. The discussion is divided into four sections: preliminary ground work, implementation, pitfalls, and evaluation and follow-up.

PRELIMINARY GROUND WORK

Ideally, preparation for instituting a campus clinical for the first time should take place the semester *before* students arrive. The logical first step is to identify the existing health-related services on the campus and the director or directors of those services, depending on the structure of the university. The services could include but not be limited to student health clinics, sexual assault services, drug education, health education, wellness programs, disability support services, and counseling services. After the directors have been identified, contact them in writing and by phone. Make sure that all services that will be interacting with students are present. To meet with all directors, you may need to set up several meetings. A face-to-face meeting is important so that discussions of the intent of the clinical and how the students can be of assistance to the unit can occur. This is critical. The multidisciplinary units need to understand that the students will be functioning as part of their team but will also have specific tasks to accomplish while they are there. The students will not be just extra bodies that the unit can use as it wishes; instead the students will have specific goals and objectives to meet when working in that unit. The multidisciplinary units also need to know that the responsibility for supervision of the students will remain with the faculty member and that directors will have input into the evaluation of the students. You can respond better to caution and resistance on the part of the health units in a face-to-face meeting than over the phone. It is important to obtain the support of these key people because they can either facilitate or block clinical experiences for students. These directors can also be helpful in identifying other units within the university that could benefit from nursing student practice. Each one should be provided with a course syllabus or at least the course objectives, required assignments, clinical days and hours, the number of students who will be functioning in each unit, and the rotation of students to different units during the semester, if applicable. The faculty should come to the meeting prepared to suggest student projects that would dovetail with the activities of the various units. Tell the units that additional student-generated projects may also be implemented under their auspices as appropriate. Once the units have been identified and the face-to-face meetings accomplished, send a confirmation letter to each unit reiterating the agreed-on schedules and projects.

What is of paramount importance is to identify a base of operations from which the students will work; in other words, a place for them to call home. At our university, home base was the community health and fitness office, the equivalent of a wellness center in other institutions. You want to avoid using the student health clinic as the home base because the main focus of that center is usually the diagnosis and treatment of illness. The main focus of the nursing course in which the students are enrolled is health promotion and disease prevention with a heavy emphasis on health education and wellness-oriented activities. The students need to be able to see the value of and opportunities available beyond the traditional role of nurse.

The next issue in initiating a campus clinical is to identify how the students can interface with the university as a whole. For this issue, the university events calendar can be of great help. The university calendar at our institution was helpful in that it identified a number of theme weeks or months throughout the academic year. For example, at the university, there is eating and body image awareness week, African American history month, women's history month, and international week. All of these event weeks or months provide opportunities for student nurses to develop health-related education projects that can be implemented during those weeks. In addition to checking the academic calendar, also consult the various health units about identified needs on the campus and how the students can be of help in the implementation of programs already developed to meet those health needs. Finally, develop suggestions for student projects as a jumping off point with additional suggestions to be added by the students themselves during the implementation of the clinical.

IMPLEMENTATION

Orientation to the Course

The next phase begins with the start of the semester and the arrival of the students at the clinical site. For this phase, plan an orientation day that includes a review of the syllabus including the course requirements, a discussion of what the students thought the clinical would be about, and an exploration of the role of the nurse in a wellness-oriented clinical site. Many students come to this type of clinical thinking they are going to be working in the student health clinic where they will be seeing sick students. They are often dismayed to discover that acute care is not the focus of the course. They need to be allowed time to digest this information and to begin to entertain the importance of nontraditional nursing roles. The faculty member needs to be committed to the clinical and genuinely enthusiastic about the learning experiences that can be obtained from such a clinical. If the faculty is not committed to the clinical and the philosophy behind it, the students will quickly pick up on the faculty member's attitude, and an opportunity for a unique learning experience will be lost.

During this initial orientation, it is also important for the faculty member to try to gain information about the students' past experiences and exposure to health education. This helps the faculty member identify and match students with the most appropriate units. Because this type of clinical requires the student to be self-directed, it is imperative that the most mature students are placed with the units that are either the most resistant to student presence or are the least organized. Students who need more structure should be placed initially in settings that have specific tasks to do.

Because our course fell during the second semester of the junior year and was only the student's second clinical experience, socialization into the profession as a whole was an ongoing process that needed to be included. One of the issues critical to the clinical was the need for confidentiality. Because these students would be interacting with other students on the campus and would be exposed to personal information, it was imperative that they realized the importance of keeping such information in confidence. To emphasize this point, each student signed a confidentiality agreement developed by the health center (Table 9–1). Even though students would not be based at the student health clinic, the confidentiality agreement was broad enough that it could also apply to other areas where students were working. In addition to the confidentiality agreement, any student who would be working with the children in the day-care center on campus needed to have a criminal background check done as mandated by state law. I obtained the forms from the state, and the students were responsible for paying the processing fee which, at the time, was $10. The

---

Table 9-1

George Mason University Student Health Center

SUBJECT: Confidentiality Statement

I understand that in the course of my clinical rotation in the George Mason University Health Center I may have access to confidential medical information concerning clients of the Center. I understand that this information has been obtained and recorded for the purpose of medical treatment. I agree that I will use this information only for the purpose of my job responsibilities, and that under no circumstances will I disclose any information about any client at the GMU Student Health Center to non-authorized personnel.

I understand that violation of this policy may be considered grounds for the termination of my clinical rotation with the Student Health Center and the course. I agree that if I have any questions about this policy, I will consult with the Administrator, Medical Director or Clinical Coordinator.

Student Signatures

Date:

Faculty Instructor Signature:

best time to complete this background check is the semester before the clinical to avoid delaying initiation of student projects with the children.

Identification of Student Projects

After the initial orientation to the course and its expectations, discuss the nursing process and how it will be used in the course. Using the nursing process, we implemented the first task. The students were told to assess the "patient" before implementing any nursing interventions. In this case, the "patient" was the university campus. To do the assessment, students obtained maps of the campus and divided it into quadrants. The students divided into groups of two or three and went out to explore the campus on foot. They were directed to look for health-related services locations, health and safety hazards, accessibility issues, and ideas for wellness projects. We encouraged students to not just look around but to go into offices, introduce themselves, and talk to personnel about their health concerns. The students were given 2 hours to accomplish the task. Because our university has a majority of students who commute rather than live on campus, this was the first time that most of the students had actually explored the campus as a whole. When they returned to home base, the students shared their observations. The students had visited everywhere on campus from the university administration offices to the power plant to student housing and food services. From this initial exploration, they began to identify the health needs of the campus community.

In their assessment of the campus, the students discovered that there were groups of people on the campus other than students who could benefit from wellness programs or health screenings. These groups included a day-care center, grounds and maintenance crews, housekeeping staff, faculty and staff, and a group of senior citizens who came to the campus for exercise and other educational programs. The students identified many more projects than could be implemented, so they prioritized their activities based on greatest need and outreach to the greatest number of people. The outcome of this process was the identification of the following activities:

- Weekly blood pressure clinics on 1 day in a stationary location and on 1 day in 1 of 4 satellite locations, which would rotate on a monthly basis.
- A health-information table tied into the university theme weeks that would rotate to various sites around the campus.
- A weekly health column in the university student newspaper.
- Health-screening services during a university-wide health fair.

In addition to the above activities in which all students would participate, individual students also developed and implemented projects that occurred on a one-time basis. Examples of these projects included

- An educational program for day-care-center children and their parents on helping children develop healthy attitudes about food
- An educational program for maintenance and grounds workers on safety for working with electricity and basic first aid for electrical burns
- An educational program on body mechanics and back safety for housekeeping staff
- A wellness assessment and an update on topics of interest to senior citizens, for instance, "What's new in osteoarthritis treatment?"
- A stress-reduction workshop featuring progressive relaxation for students.

In each of the above examples, one or two students took responsibility for researching, planning, and implementing the various projects. Box 9-1 contains examples of on-campus issues for students to discuss.

Box 9-1   Learning Exercise for Faculty Use

Campus Issues

You are staffing the health-education table on campus. A student approaches you and tells you she is worried about her roommate. She thinks her roommate has an eating disorder. Her roommate spends a lot of time in the bathroom, and the student thinks she has heard her throwing up. The roommate denies any problems with eating or being sick. What do you do?

Your student is staffing the rotating blood pressure clinic. She takes the blood pressure of a maintenance worker. The blood pressure reading is 186/104. What do you do?

Perhaps where the students were the most creative was with the health information table. They coined the name "NursEnergy" for their clinical group, made a big table banner, and used it to set up their health information table each week. They also used the same name to identify themselves in the health column in the student newspaper (Table 9–2). After several weeks, students on campus began to identify who this group of students were and to approach them with health questions. It was a rewarding and meaningful experience for all involved.

Use of Clinical Time

This particular clinical course was a 4-semester-hour course. Using a 3:1 hour lab ratio, the students were in clinical for 6 hours, 2 days per week for a total of 12 hours per week.

As previously stated, a number of on-campus units were identified as having health-related services. Because it was not feasible for all students to rotate through all sites, I divided up the sites and assigned students by their interest or expertise. Optimally, students were to have experience in at least three different health-related activities

Table 9-2

Ask a Nurse
by NursEnergy

NursEnergy is a group of clinical students from the College of Nursing & Health Science. Our purpose is to answer your health questions through this weekly column as a service to the GMU community. We will also be staffing a health information table Tuesdays and Thursdays throughout the semester. Look for us in the SUB I or SUB II lobbies. It doesn't hurt to ask!

Q: How many calories should I be eating each day?

A: We tend to think of calories as "things to eat" when they actually are a measurement of the energy we get from the food we eat. Our bodies use this energy for several processes, including cell and organ functioning, maintenance of normal body temperature, physical activity, and growth.

The number of daily calories necessary for the best health and functioning of your body is determined by several things: body size, sex, age, and activity level. Larger bodies need more calories. Males need more calories than females. After about age 19, calorie requirements decline with age. The more active you are, the more calories you will require.

Since we don't know your age, let's use a hypothetical GMU student as an example: If she's 24, moderately active and weighs 128 pounds, she will need approximately 2,200 calories per day. If he's 24, moderately active and weighs 160 pounds, 2,900 calories will meet his requirements.

To determine your personal calorie needs, visit the NursEnergy Information table.

Q: How much sleep should I be getting each night?

A: Human beings spend approximately one-third of their lives asleep. Although many people believe eight hours of sleep per night is necessary, research has found some people need more, and others can function well with considerably less. Infants require the largest amounts of sleep, as do growing children and adolescents during their growth spurts (males up to age 20), because protein synthesis occurs most readily during sleep.

Sleep relieves tension and conserves energy. Sleep is a protective function, which allows for repair and recovery of tissues following activity. Without adequate sleep, we become irritable, anxious, depressed, and apathetic, and we suffer from general body malaise and lethargy. If you are feeling fine, you're probably getting enough sleep. You can cheat yourself occasionally, but constant sleep loss can be dangerous.

Do you have a question for Ask A Nurse? Contact us c/o Broadside, Room 253A, SUB I, MSN 2C5, 4400 University Dr., Fairfax, VA 22030.

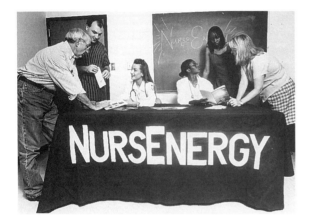

on the campus, the faculty blocked out those 2 hours per week to provide direct supervision of the students and counted it as on-campus time. The students received 2 hours payback time from a clinical day of their choice.

Finally, a clinical conference was held once a week for 2 hours so that students could update the group on individual activities, discuss problems, and brainstorm problem-solving strategies. The clinical conference time also allowed the faculty to provide for group guidance, give reminders regarding deadlines, request additional services from the university, and assess the progress of the clinical as a whole. The once-a-week format worked better than trying to have a clinical conference each clinical day.

during the semester. A variety of experiences would keep the students from becoming bored with activities, such as blood pressure screening, that are repetitive. The students needed to develop and implement both group and individual teaching projects as part of the course objectives. In addition, some of the units on campus had specific requests for the minimum length of time they felt each student needed to spend in the particular unit. Therefore, we set up a rotation grid to provide a visual tracking system for the students (Table 9–3). Each student and each unit received a copy. The clinical group also developed and distributed a phone tree of all students and the instructor.

Students were also required to keep a time log to document their use of clinical time when they were not directly in client contact (Table 9–4). I allowed use of some clinical time for library research, gathering equipment, and obtaining written teaching aids from various agencies for the development of teaching projects. Students used clinical time to develop surveys, questionnaires, and other tools to assist them in their health education projects (Tables 9–5, 9–6, 9–7, and 9–8).

Some projects required that the students be available outside of clinical hours. Students who could be flexible took on those assignments in coordination with the faculty who was also either available on-site with students or available by pager. An example of this was the immunization clinic. This experience was designed to provide an opportunity for students to practice the skill of giving injections as well as educating the student clients about the immunizations. The clinic hours, however, were on a different day than the regular clinical. Because the site was

Supervision of Students

Each clinical day the instructor needs to make "rounds," visiting the students at their different locations. I would set up times to meet with at least three to four students one-on-one each clinical day for an extended period to discuss their projects, concerns, problems, and frustrations. It also gave me a chance to see if the individual student was grasping the philosophy and intent of the course. To help with this, each student kept a journal of activities, thoughts, and feelings and how well he or she was meeting course objectives. An example of one student's journal entry is provided here.

 Today I participated for one final time at the NursEnergy table. It is Victim's Rights week, and our concentration was on women's health issues. We didn't get the opportunity to talk to too many people today, but we did get to enjoy a self-defense demonstration.

It has been a different learning experience than I expected at the table. I truly believe we gained more scientific knowledge about the topics we covered, which included a large spectrum of topics. It was a vehicle by which we also learned what topics are most important to the GMU community. As I have stated before in my clinical logs, the topics don't always include those presented at the table. As a health practitioner, the public expects you to be knowledgeable in many areas that concern medicine, nursing, public health, and education.

After having our clinical conference in the afternoon, we adjourned for the day.

Clinical time: 9 am to 3:30 pm.

Table 9-3

Clinical Rotation Grid

UNIT

WEEK	HEALTH EDUCATION	COMMUNITY HEALTH & FITNESS	DRUG EDUCATION	SEXUAL ASSAULT SERVICES	STUDENT HEALTH CLINIC	CHILD DEVELOPMENT CENTER	COUNSELING CENTER	BLACK PEER COUNSELING
1								
2								
3								
4								
5								
6								
7								
8								
9								
10								
11								
12								
13								
14								

Table 9-4

Student Time Log

Name:

CLINICAL SITE:

DATE	ACTIVITY	TIME SPENT	RUNNING TOTAL

Table 9-5 — Health Promotion Survey

The Black Peer Counseling Program and the George Mason University (GMU) Nursing School are involved in a joint venture to promote health education projects designed to benefit the black student population here at GMU. We have developed this survey so that you can inform us about the health promotion issues that are of interest to you. Please place a check mark beside the issues that interest you.

Health Promotion Issues:

- ☐ 1. High Blood Pressure
- ☐ 2. Body Fat Analysis
- ☐ 3. Cholesterol Testing
- ☐ 4. Dental Care/Oral Cancer
- ☐ 5. Nutrition (Basic) Eating Habits
- ☐ 6. Low-Fat Recipes
- ☐ 7. Smoking Cessation
- ☐ 8. Breast Self-Examination
- ☐ 9. Diseases
- ☐ 10. Diabetes
- ☐ 11. Learning Types
- ☐ 12. Depression
- ☐ 13. Time Management
- ☐ 14. Stress Management
- ☐ 15. Assertiveness Training
- ☐ 16. Dealing with Death/Loss or Divorce
- ☐ 17. Self-Esteem
- ☐ 18. Sickle Cell Anemia
- ☐ 19. Heart Disease
- ☐ 20. Testicular Self-Examination
- ☐ 21. First Aid Information
- ☐ 22. Financial Costs
- ☐ 23. Health Insurance
- ☐ 24. Other (please specify) _____

Fitness and Exercise:

- ☐ 25. Weight Management
- ☐ 26. Aerobics
- ☐ 27. Weight (Lifting) Training

Child Care Issues:

- ☐ 28. Child Health-Care Issues
- ☐ 29. Pregnancy
- ☐ 30. Raising Healthy Children

Class Status:
- ☐ 1. Freshman
- ☐ 2. Sophomore
- ☐ 3. Junior
- ☐ 4. Senior
- ☐ 5. Other

Age:
- ☐ 1. 17 or younger
- ☐ 2. 18–22
- ☐ 3. 23–25
- ☐ 4. 25 or older

Race:
- ☐ 1. Native-American
- ☐ 2. Black
- ☐ 3. White
- ☐ 4. Hispanic
- ☐ 5. Asian
- ☐ 6. Other

Sex:
- ☐ 1. Male
- ☐ 2. Female

Marital Status:
- ☐ 1. Single
- ☐ 2. Married
- ☐ 3. Divorced

Academic Major: _____

Would you be interested in a lifestyle assessment to determine your health status and potential risk factors?   ☐ Yes   ☐ No

Table 9-6

Health- and Wellness-promotion Education Projects

Based on the results obtained from the health-promotion survey, the following health-promotion issues will be presented in the Black Peer Counseling Office.

1. Blood Pressure Screening	Feb. 20, Feb. 21	11:00 am – 3:00 pm 11:00 am – 3:00 pm
2. Body Fat Analysis & Weight Management	Feb. 27, Feb. 29	11:00 am – 3:00 pm 9:00 am – 12 noon
3. Nutrition & Cholesterol Testing Information	March 5, March 7	11:00 am – 3:00 pm 9:00 am – 12 noon
4. Time Management & Stress Management	March 21	9:00 am – 12 noon
5. Breast Self-exam & Endometriosis	April 2, April 4	11:00 am – 3:00 pm 9:00 am – 12 noon
6. Dental/Oral Cancer	April 9	10:00 am – 2:00 pm
7. Raising Healthy Children	April 11	9:00 am – 12 noon
8. Financial Cost (medical & mental)	April 16	9:00 am – 2:00 pm
9. Weight Lifting & Aerobics	April 18	9:00 am – 12 noon
10. Sickle Cell Anemia	April 23	9:00 am – 2:00 pm
11. Testicular Self-exam	April 25	9:00 am – 12 noon

Another entry:

 Today I will be returning the stress game to the Woodburn Clinic in Annandale. I have attached a copy of the note of thanks to...of the Woodburn Clinic. She has stated that we (GMU Nursing) are welcome to borrow the game any time. Her phone number and the clinic's are included for your future reference.

Tomorrow Regina and I will be attending the BSE facilitator presentation at the American Cancer Society in Vienna, VA. We will then return to campus in the afternoon.

Friday I will have the opportunity to spend the morning with the nurse practitioner in the GMU Health Clinic. Next Tuesday, I spend time with Molly in the morning completing part 2 of the biofeedback clinic. I will continue to work on my final article for the BROADSIDE on the subject of chromium.

It's hard to believe this semester is almost over. So much has been gained. And there is so much to learn. Thanks for being there. We couldn't have had a better instructor. Your guidance and patience set a wonderful standard for our future in nursing.

The journals were not graded, so students were encouraged to be honest about their feelings. There would be no negative consequences for expressing how they felt. The journals were collected every 2 weeks on the 2nd clinical day at the clinical conference. The instructor would read them, make comments in the journal, and make his or her own notes. The journals would then be returned on the first day of the following week. The journals give insight into students who were struggling, those who were being productive, and those who were not being productive. The instructor could then appropriately

Table 9-7 Eating Pattern Awareness Survey

Interested in how you think about food and your body? So are we. Fill out this survey form and help us get an idea of how college students feel about food and fat.
Please circle one best answer.

Sex: Male   Female   **Age Group:**   15–20   21–25   26–30   31–35   36+

How much are you above or below your recommended body weight?			Are you happy with the way your body looks?			
Within range	Within 5 lb	More than 5 lb	Never	Sometimes	Often	Always
0	1	2	3	2	1	0

How much do you think about what you eat?				Do you feel comfortable eating with other people?			
Never	Sometimes	Often	Always	Never	Sometimes	Often	Always
0	1	2	3	3	2	1	0

Do you hide how much or how little you eat from others?				How often do you eat alone?			
Never	Sometimes	Often	Always	Never	Sometimes	Often	Always
0	1	2	3	0	0	2	3

How often do you use a laxative?					Do you think you answered this form truthfully?			
Never	Sometimes	Monthly	Weekly	Daily	Never	Sometimes	Often	Always
0	1	2	3	4	3	2	1	0

Scoring: Add the numbers up under your answers. A score of 5+ suggests that you are at risk for developing problematic eating habits.

For more information call the Counseling Center at 555-0000.

(Developed by Meg Trainor, student. (1995, February); Fairfax: GMU College of Nursing and Health Science.)

Table 9–8 Healthy Living Pilot Survey

To: Members of the Health Education and the Physical Fitness Program for Older Adults (HEP)

Purpose: To identify your health concerns and interests

Sex: ☐ M ☐ F   Age: _____   Race: _____

1. What specific time and day (Monday–Friday) could you attend a program of interest?

2. Place a check by any of the following health issues you would like addressed such as:

- ☐ Diabetes
- ☐ Hypertension (High Blood Pressure)
- ☐ Heart Disease
- ☐ Arthritis
- ☐ Smoking Cessation
- ☐ Nutrition/Cholesterol Reduction
- ☐ Dealing with Loss
- ☐ Divorce
- ☐ Living Alone

- ☐ Cancer (types) _____
- ☐ Body Fat Analysis
- ☐ Osteoporosis
- ☐ Respiratory Problems
- ☐ Exercise
- ☐ Stress Reduction
- ☐ Bereavement
- ☐ Other (please specify) _____

(From Gibson Erhunmwunse, student. Fairfax: GMU College of Nursing and Health Science.)

schedule one-on-one meetings with the students. We also blocked out time to attend student educational presentations when they were implemented. Box 9-2 provides you with two scenarios to use with your students.

> **Box 9-2** Learning Exercise for Faculty Use
>
> ### Critical Thinking Scenarios
>
> Your student is assigned to the child development center. He is teaching a group of 4-year-olds about good touch/bad touch. In the course of the presentation, one child asks, "What if your daddy touches you there, is that OK?" What do you do?
>
> Your student is screening tuberculosis (TB) skin-test results. A university student presents with an obvious positive reaction. She states that she is in this country on a student visa and is afraid she will be deported because she skin-tested positive. She begins to cry. What do you do?

Problems and Pitfalls

As with any new endeavor, there were unanticipated problems in both planning and implementation that we could not anticipate. One of the early pitfalls was the need to have the criminal background check completed prior to working at the day-care center. It takes about 2 weeks for the applications to be processed, and because some students are on very tight budgets, even a $10 fee was a hardship. As a result, it took almost a month to get all students processed. It is much better to identify the students during the preceding semester so that they will be ready to go on day 1.

Another pitfall was the health column in the student newspaper. Because the paper was run by students, I as a faculty member had no influence on the acceptance of a health column. It was only through the efforts of a particularly articulate and enthusiastic student that the column became a reality. Because the editors of the newspaper change every year as do the students in my clinical, the health column cannot be counted on as a viable project. You need to go back to square one each time you teach the clinical. One possible inroad would be to

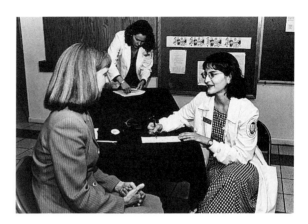

develop a relationship with the faculty advisor for the student newspaper. This person would have more influence with the student editors than you would.

Another situation was being able to identify the student who was not performing well early in the semester. Because virtually all of the students were working with individuals who were not nurses, these individuals needed guidelines as to what was acceptable or unacceptable student behavior. For example, one student spent a significant amount of clinical time attending workshops under the guise of research for her own presentation. Each time I checked with the unit director, I was told the student was off-site doing research. It took me awhile to catch on to what was meant by "research." I then developed a guide for each unit, identifying the nature of clinical time for students and what would be acceptable activities during that time (Table 9–9).

Perhaps the biggest concern in setting up this clinical was the reluctance of some units to participate. Most of the unit personnel, if they had ever worked with students at all, had worked with students as preceptors. This type of role was perceived as a burden by the personnel who already had full calendars. This problem was counteracted by assuring the personnel that the instructor was to be the student supervisor and that they would be contributing to student evaluation but not totally responsible for it. The units were also reassured that the instructor would deal with any problems that arose with students.

Other personnel could not see the relevance of having a nursing student. In other words, they could not see why a nurse would be involved in the activities of their particular unit. I needed to spend considerable time with the units

> **Table 9-9**
>
> ## Clinical Time Usage Guidelines
>
> The students are assigned to your unit for a period of 3–4 weeks with the exception of Black Peer Counseling and the Counseling Center where 1–2 students will be assigned for the entire semester. The students spend 12 hours a week in clinical, 6 hrs on Tuesday and 6 hrs on Thursday. Following are suggestions of valid uses of clinical time:
>
> 1. Students should check in with the unit coordinator each clinical day. If the student will not be on site on any given clinical day, he or she must contact the unit coordinator by phone.
> 2. Students may use clinical time to research teaching projects at the library, or off-site at various agencies. However, at least 1 clinical day each week should be spent in the unit.
> 3. Students should have direct contact with those who use your services at least twice during their assignment to your unit.
> 4. Students can be used to help you complete health-related projects your unit is producing, but their entire clinical time should not be used for this purpose because each student will have course goals that they need to meet as well.
> 5. Students may need to be away from your unit periodically to participate in other clinical activities. In such cases, the student(s) will notify you of the dates and times they will be gone.
> 6. If at any time you feel that the students are not being productive or using their clinical time inappropriately, please feel free to page me.
> 7. This clinical requires students to be self-directed and capable of independent actions. If you feel that any of the students assigned to your unit is incapable of such behavior, please notify me and I will work with the student in this area.
> 8. Students will be keeping a log of their clinical time. Feel free to ask to see these logs at any time.

involved defining the scope of nursing practice and discussing the various roles nurses play in the whole healthcare arena. Like many people not in the health field, the image that is held of nursing is still that of the bedside, acute-care nurse. After the clinical began, a continuous reinforcement of the contributions nurses make in different health arenas was needed to minimize resistance.

Another problem was the length of time students would spend in any given unit. Several units had specific requests or projects to be implemented, and the length of time a student committed varied from unit to unit. The time commitments ranged from 2 weeks to the entire semester. An example of semester-long commitments was a student who took on the project of developing a biweekly series of health education programs for African-American students based on the health risks for that particular ethnic group. Another student committed to learning how to use the biofeedback equipment in the counseling center and then designed a training manual for other students who would follow her in that site. She also prepared and taught several stress reduction workshops using the biofeedback equipment. Students assigned to a specific unit for the whole semester also participated in one or two ongoing weekly activities so that they had exposure to several different types of education or assessment and screening activities.

The timing of some of the projects was also problematic. Because some of the target groups met on days other than clinical days, students needed to work out times that would fit their schedule, my schedule, and the schedule of the target group. This limited the participation of some students who did not have the flexibility of others and also limited some of the projects because of my lack of availability. The best way to deal with this is to identify the project times when the initial projects are being identified and prioritized.

Another situation arose concerning one of the course objectives, which mandated that each student complete a family assessment. Originally it was thought that students from the disabilities support service would be an excellent group to draw on. What we found, however, was that this group of students was fiercely independent and did not feel they could benefit from such an assessment. An idea that came to me during the semester, but I was unable to initiate, was to put an appeal into the disabilities support services newsletter asking students to volunteer to be interviewed as a way of providing a service to the nursing students. They could help to educate the nursing students about living with disabilities and how they and their families have adapted.

The family assessment objective was the most difficult objective to meet. We accomplished it through interviews with the senior citizen group on campus. Although the students were able to obtain basic information, they did not make home visits, which would have enriched the assessment tremendously.

All in all, most of the problems that arose were resolved in a timely fashion. Afterwards, these pitfalls as well as suggested recommendations were put into a guide for subsequent faculty who would be involved in this clinical.

Evaluation and Follow-up

At the end of the clinical, it is important for the faculty to close the experience by writing letters of thanks and evaluating the program. Write thank-you letters to the head of each unit where students were placed as well as to each individual who helped in the supervision of students. The letters to the heads of the units should include the contributions of the individual staff members because this information could possibly be used for merit raises or other types of recognition. In addition, survey all the units about the unit's perception of the clinical experience (Table 9–10).

Table 9-10

Unit Evaluation of the Campus Clinical

Please fill out your perception of the campus clinical for the College of Nursing. Return completed forms to Lucy Boland, RNC, MSN, Faculty Instructor, MSN 3C4, College of Nursing and Health Science via campus mail. Your comments are important to us and will be used as we make revisions to the course. Thank you for your assistance.

1. Describe how the nursing students were either an asset or barrier to the functioning of your unit.

2. Was the length of time the student(s) spent in your area sufficient to meet your goals? If not, what length of time would you suggest?

3. Was the faculty member readily available to you? Do you feel she spent enough time with the student(s)?

4. How do you see nursing students functioning in your unit in future clinical rotations?

5. Other comments, recommendations.

Last, the students themselves should evaluate the clinical and be given the opportunity to suggest additional opportunities or to identify problem areas. Most schools have a standardized evaluation form for students. We used this standardized form (computer generated with a Likert scale) and a form that would solicit a narrative assessment of the clinical experience (Table 66). The narrative form provided more concrete information than the university's computerized generic form. The narrative form also allowed students to make suggestions for additional activities for subsequent clinical groups.

Because this clinical was unstructured and because the students were interfacing with other health discipline individuals, the biggest challenge was helping the students see these health-related activities as legitimate and important parts of nursing practice. For example, during eating and body-image awareness week on campus, the counseling center had already put together a self-assessment to identify students at risk for anorexia or bulimia. The center also had assembled educational materials on eating disorders. The nursing students who were going to participate with the counseling center were at a loss as to what they could do that was different and related to nursing. What we came up with together was a handout that discussed the physiological changes and problems that occur as a result of an eating disorder. This dovetailed nicely with the counseling center's psychological approach.

In conclusion, using a college campus as a clinical rotation site can be a unique, productive, and service-oriented experience for both students and faculty alike. It involves a lot of preliminary planning, from contacting campus offices and meeting with directors of various health-related units to identifying potential student projects. Once the semester has begun, the faculty needs to make a major time commitment to socializing students into a nontraditional nursing role. The faculty needs to continue close contact with the units where students are placed to assess for potential problems as well as to socialize the personnel of those units to the nontraditional role of the nurse. Keeping close contact with students is critical because the clinical setting is unstructured, and students will need assistance with managing their time in a productive way that meets the course objectives. Last, evaluation and follow-up are also critical to the successful implementation of such a clinical. Identifying what did and did not work is critical to refining and increasing the effectiveness of the clinical experience. Acknowledging the assistance of the various units on campus that were involved in the clinical helps to maintain good working relationships.

This type of clinical will help students expand their horizons with regard to the role of the nurse. It will help them develop their written and verbal communication skills, their assessment skills, and their teaching skills. It can also be a lot of fun!

References

American Health Consultants, Inc. (1994). College HIV rate holds steady, but risk of exposure remains high. AIDS Alert 9(11), 153–156.

Conyne, R, et al. (1994). Applying primary prevention precepts to campus substance abuse programs. J Counsel Devel 72(6), 603–608.

Georgiou, C, et al. (1997). Among young adults, college students and graduates practiced more healthful habits and made more healthful food choices than did nonstudents. J Am Diet Assoc 97(7), 754–759.

Haspel, J (1998). Social pressure, not peer pressure, leads students to drink. The Brown University Child and Adolescent Behavior Letter, 14(9), 1–3.

Heatherton, T, et al. (1995). Body weight, dieting, and eating disorder symptoms among college students, 1982 to 1992. Am J Psychiatry 152(11), 1623–1629.

Ho, G, et al. (1998). Natural history of cervicovaginal papillomavirus infection in young women. N Engl J Med 338(7), 423–428.

McNair, L, et al. (1998). Self-esteem, gender, and alcohol use: relationships with HIV risk perception and behaviors in college students. J Sex Marital Ther 24(1), 29–36.

Mangweth, B, et al. (1995). Bulimia nervosa in two cultures: a comparison of Austrian and American college students. Int J Eat Disord 17(4), 403–412.

Maticka-Tyndale, E, et al. (1998). Casual sex on spring break: Intentions and behaviors of Canadian students. J Sex Res 35(3), 254–264.

Miller, J. (1997). Clinic nurses: confronting campus alcohol use on the frontline. J Am Coll Health 45(5), 205–208.

Minoia, J. (1996). Attitudes toward condom use among female college students. J N Y State Nurses Assoc 27(3), 4–7.

Prince, A, et al. (1998). Sexual behaviors and safer sex practices of college students on a commuter campus. J Am Coll Health 47(1), 11-21.

Roehrig, H, & Range, L. (1995). Recklessness, depression, and reasons for living in predicting suicidality in college students. J Youth & Adolescence 24(6), 723-729.

Seymour, M, et al. (1997). Inappropriate dieting behaviors and related lifestyle factors in young adults: Are college students different? J Nutr Edu 29(1), 21.

Wall, A, et al. (1998). Alcohol outcome expectancies, attitudes toward drinking and the theory of planned behavior. J Stud Alcohol 59(4), 409-419.

CHAPTER 10
Teaching Students in a Community HIV/AIDS Network

Loretta Brush Normile

Learning Objectives

1) Identify appropriate learning experiences for students in a community-based HIV/AIDS network.
2) Specify the phases in establishment of a community-based HIV/AIDS network.
3) Discuss how to enhance collaboration with health professionals in the community.
4) Discuss the supervision required to assure safe student practice in community-based settings.
5) Identify teaching strategies to promote student learning.
6) Compare and contrast the scope of faculty practice in community-based HIV/AIDS settings and in traditional settings.

This chapter tells the story of the interactive, creative process of establishing and developing a community-based HIV/AIDS clinical placement for George Mason University's (GMU) College of Nursing and Health Science. Following the transformation of our traditional nursing curriculum to a community-based curriculum, there was a search for appropriate junior-level community-based settings that would give our students the opportunity to practice health promotion, disease prevention, therapeutic communication, and health assessment. This quest provided the impetus for the evolutionary process that has transformed one clinical placement into the present clinical network of HIV/AIDS community-based practice.

The partnership that is fundamental to this clinical experience is a venture between the Inova's Juniper Program in Northern Virginia and the College of Nursing and Health Science at GMU, Fairfax, Virginia. The Juniper Program as a clinical site offers many advantages. It is an Area Education and Training Center for HIV/AIDS. It is a well-established training program for health professionals and offers state-of-the-art information on managing HIV-infected clients, skills building in the care and prevention of HIV/AIDS, and experiential training through a variety of learning modules.

The students who take the course, and their clients, are also key to this partnership; they are the journeyers who are exploring firsthand community health and the approaches to preventing HIV and AIDS, or caring for those infected or at risk for HIV disease. The partnership offers students and clients a learner-centered approach in the community with an emphasis on experiential learning and critical reflection.

My story begins in Fairfax on that first clinical day. It was a sunny but cold February morning, and I was thrilled to begin this new community-based experience with the INOVA Juniper Program. As I entered the familiar yellow brick building, a place I had come to many times for HIV/AIDS training, continuing education, and resources, I felt fortunate to have such a setting for my students. I was viewed as a colleague by the staff there. I also had educational background and expertise in the field of HIV/AIDS and was certain the community health course objectives would easily be met at this clinical placement. As I entered the training room, the junior nursing students were just arriving, and the education coordinator was setting out fresh bagels, hot coffee, and tea for us. The students told me later they felt so welcomed and nurtured that morning. They perceived a learning climate that was supportive from the first day.

Aside from the usual orientation activities to a new site, those first 2 clinical days gave the students an overview of HIV/AIDS and an introduction to the existing training program. This included content deemed to be essential for their learning (Table 10–1). As we began the clinical rotation that first semester, it seemed relatively simple. My 10 nursing students would be scheduled by the education coordinator to complete the very same modules that were set up for the professional health caregivers. The students were placed in the community to work with individuals, families, and small groups. They would interact with clients who were at risk for, or infected with, the HIV virus. These included children, adolescents, women, and men. Students would care for vulnerable groups comprised of homosexuals, heterosexuals, substance abusers, and hemophiliacs. With agency and faculty assistance, students would rotate through several settings such as homes, respite day care, clinics, emergency shelters, counseling and testing centers, and schools. These settings would give the students the opportunity to see and care for clients where they live, work, and play, and across a continuum of care.

Although all went well those first 2 days, the next clinical day presented more of a challenge for me as the

Table 10-1

Essential Knowledge for Students in an HIV/AIDS Community-based Setting

- Values clarification
- Personal feelings and attitudes about HIV/AIDS
- Basic epidemiology about HIV/AIDS
- Compliance with treatment protocols
- Pathophysiology of HIV and opportunistic infections
- Nursing management of HIV
- Universal precautions with blood borne pathogens
- Transmission of HIV
- Prevention measures/safer sex practices
- HIV testing/pretest, posttest, and counseling
- Risk assessment
- Care of the HIV-positive and AIDS client
- Antiretroviral therapy and adherence
- Wellness and health maintenance of persons living with HIV
- Long-term survivorship

students began their rotations. When I arrived that 3rd clinical day, the staff looked puzzled. What was I doing there this particular day, they asked? With the clinical training program they currently had in place, arrangements were made for the "trainee." The trainee arrived at the site with an emphasis on experiential learning but with no hands-on activities. All "training" was coordinated by the Juniper Program. What I had in mind for our students (and was sure I had communicated) was a collaborative relationship between student, faculty, and site preceptor with access to individuals, families, and small groups for health promotion, disease prevention, therapeutic communication, and nursing assessment opportunities. Soon, assigning the students became complicated. The days and times of some experiences varied from our clinical hours and were based on the availability of the training sites.

IDENTIFYING APPROPRIATE LEARNING EXPERIENCES

Accommodating 10 nursing students, one at each agency or site, quickly strained the agency's limited personnel and physical resources. The education coordinator was overwhelmed with placing 10 students in the limited openings of the various learning modules (Table 10–2). This made it increasingly difficult for the Office of HIV Services to carry out its primary mission of HIV/AIDS training for licensed nurses, doctors, dentists, counselors, and social workers. What resulted was not enough clinical experiences for my students. This problem would have been prevented by better communication between the host agency and the College of Nursing and Health Science. An additional, comparable site rotation could have been added at that time.

In the days that followed, I spent much time looking beyond the Juniper Program for valid experiences to fill clinical hours each week. I first needed to identify other resources and resource people. It was necessary to determine what was out there at every level of the community. I perused community resource manuals on HIV/AIDS. It was clear the HIV Services program was central to my HIV/AIDS rotation, but there were agencies providing other services in the community that could prove relevant in the student experience with HIV/AIDS. Community agencies that serve specific populations and deal with infectious disease, incarceration, substance abuse, hemophilia, and juveniles were explored. Several of these agencies had the potential to provide students with access to groups at high risk for HIV/AIDS. But most could accommodate only one student at a time. From this I was able to develop several modules: a substance abuse module, a case management/clinical studies module, respite child care module for HIV-positive clients, and an adolescent prevention module. One agency, a juvenile emergency shelter, had such a great need for HIV/AIDS education for their juveniles that 6 years later, students are still teaching about sexually transmitted diseases, HIV, and safer sex practices to this highly vulnerable population. The other faculty-eveloped learning modules are still functional and working well for both students and agency.

During this initial experience, I found scheduling and coordination of clinical experiences extremely time-consuming. I still do. I occasionally find myself trying to develop an alliance with a site that later proves not to be a good fit. I believe most clinical faculty have found themselves in that situation. While developing a network of experiences, you have the opportunity to determine your "fit" before you become involved in a teaching-learning partnership. I find most agencies are open to this. The following box will help you educate your commmunity.

Table 10-2

Examples of Learning Modules

- Adolescent management
- Case management
- Case management of clients in clinical HIV research protocols*
- Hemophiliac clinic*
- Home health care
- HIV counseling and testing
- Mental health
- Nutritional care*
- Pediatric management
- Palliative care/hospice*
- Prevention programs for youth*
- Respite child care for parents with AIDS*
- Substance abuse*

*Faculty-developed modules

Box 10-1   Learning Exercise for Faculty Use

Community Activity

Contact an agency in your community, and work with them to develop a workshop for persons living in the community with HIV/AIDS. Utilize a discussion format or a panel rather than a lecture.

Table 10-3

Faculty-developed Modules

- Juvenile detention/probation centers
- Jails and prisons
- Comprehensive addiction treatment centers
- Hospices
- Shelters
- Home-health-care agencies
- Nutritional programs that deliver meals to AIDS clients and families
- Voluntary agencies that service HIV/AIDS clients and families
- Street outreach prevention programs
- Respite care programs for AIDS families
- Counseling and testing centers
- HIV/AIDS clinics

As the junior-level clinical continues to develop, the clinical network continues to expand. Currently, the HIV/AIDS network allows me to coordinate one-to-one service learning experiences for students in dozens of area community agencies. Collaboratively with the faculty member, each student selects several modules for HIV education, clinical training, and mentoring from the Office of HIV Services' original modules. I have expanded these to include modules on substance-abuse treatment, jails, and HIV/AIDS outreach programs among others (Table 10–3). This approach allows students to gain access to culturally diverse and vulnerable populations, gaining skills in provision of care for and education of HIV infected and uninfected clients.

PHASES IN ESTABLISHMENT OF AN HIV NETWORK

I found the phases in establishment of a community-based HIV/AIDS network parallel to Norwood's (1998) phases of the consultation process. These steps include gaining entry, engagement and evaluation, and disengagement, if or when necessary. I find initial entry into a potential network setting to be a time of relationship building and defining. I scan the environment to determine if this setting would be a fit between the students' needs and the agency's interests, services, and needs. This is done through indirect observation and informal meetings (even over lunch or networking at conferences). These meetings should include familiarization of the agency mission and goals. The Internet, publicity, brochures, and news reports have also helped me to gain valuable insight into the agency's needs, values, and personality. If this initial phase ends in a mutual decision for students to enter the setting, the process of identifying mutual wants begins, and a formal contract is made with the College of Nursing and Health Science.

The process of psychological entry involves engaging the agency. It is important to be able to describe exactly how the outcomes of the student experience can benefit the agency. I feel a need to establish my credibility and promote a sense of trust on the part of the community agency. This is an important aspect because it leads to future problem solving and development of mutual respect and cooperation between the students and the agency. I stay visible by being an active participant on agency committees and task forces, periodically reviewing proposals, and volunteering with them occasionally.

I do a formative evaluation of the relationship between students and agency as the experience is unfolding. Students and key agency staff sit down and informally discuss how the experience is going for them. This permits on-the-spot or mid-semester changes and greatly increases the likelihood that the alliance with the agency will be successful. At the end of the course, I arrange a luncheon for the students and all the agency preceptors and key contact people. Feedback is shared in an informal atmosphere of collegiality. Because this is an activity that takes place at the end of the semester, it is a rather joyous occasion for the students. It offers a chance to get closure and celebrate their key contacts and preceptors. Each year this activity gets better and better as the network continues to solidify. Agency members report that it is a time for networking for them with other agencies as well.

I find planning, revision, and evaluation of the modules to be ongoing. Variables such as agency personnel changes, the changing health-care environment, financial dynamics, and census changes are challenges that I face every semester. Also, gaining access to an HIV/AIDS community agency requires administration-level sanctioning of the partnership with the nursing program and student-client activities.

The collaboration with health professionals and members of community groups is a distinctive feature of the design, implementation, and evaluation of this clinical experience. As this network continues to evolve, I seek consultation and guidance from many of the nurses and other health professionals directly involved in HIV/AIDS prevention and care in the community. Many are now contributing to the teaching-learning experiences in this clinical network. Communication, supervision, and scope-of-practice issues are addressed at each site, and the related experiences evolve with examples of what is working, as well as what is failing to work. Specific learning experiences and teaching strategies for application of primary care knowledge and skills are described. I frequently find the students' journal entries give valuable personal insights and practical information relating to particular agencies and experiences. I request permission to photocopy and share those insights with the appropriate person(s) at the agencies whenever possible. I find myself presenting information, role modeling, and providing expertise and leadership to students and agencies (Norwood 1998). But unlike the consulting relationship, collaboration here takes place between myself and the agency on behalf of the students. Tasks and activities of each step have to be implemented with flexibility to allow for the unique characteristics of the agency or experience. If they aren't, important information about the experience or intervention opportunities would result in problems with that experience. As a relationship with an agency and member progresses, new information and opportunities within the agency emerge. I find myself in a continuous process of assessing, planning, implementing, and evaluating to develop a trusting relationship with the agency contact persons or mentors, the staff, and the clients. The phases of this process may overlap, requiring a back-and-forth approach. As problems occur, some steps may need to be repeated to resolve the problem.

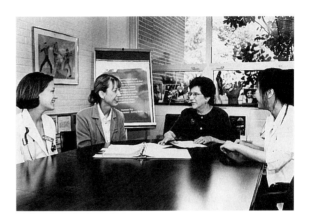

Occasionally, a site and its related experiences fail to produce expected educational outcomes despite problem-solving attempts. Sense of timing is a key factor. This is a time to establish or change maintenance supports, engage in relationship review, realize psychodynamics, and achieve closure (Norwood 1998, p 228).

Disengagement can trigger a plethora of emotions for faculty, students, and agency staff. It is possible to see dependency behaviors, retreat, passivity, or rising conflict on the part of any or all involved in the educational experience, including the clients. The question you must ask is if the timing of the disengagement from a particular agency or experience is crucial to the success of the teaching-learning experience, or are there other issues and needs that should be considered? I believe the door should always be left open for future collaboration. Initially, there may be no opportunities to see the consequences of disengagement. Formal post-termination follow-up as well as informal follow-up activities through professional endeavors, mutual colleagues, and networking can be worked into disengagement plans. It is crucial for students to see that learning can occur in both positive and negative situations. The learning that occurs from an unsuccessful relationship or partnership can increase the possibility of success in future liaisons.

Collaboration with Health Professionals

Collaboration with health professionals is a distinguishing feature of the experience. In addition, students reap great benefits from networking opportunities that will greatly enhance their entry into professional practice.

The course is taught in a flexible manner to allow for individual learning needs, career goals, and past experiences. The faculty-student relationship is more of a partnership, and at times, a collegial relationship, wherein the clinical faculty member facilitates learning experiences that vary from student to student. Students take an active role in determining the initial clinical experiences and activities within the context of the course objectives.

In addition to regularly planned conference times, there are many daily interactions in the settings between students, myself, and agency staff. These interactions concern questions and issues that arise in the student experience. For instance, after a day at an HIV counseling and testing site, students wanted to discuss sexual issues that came up in their experience with the patients and clients; these issues are difficult for even the most sophisticated counselor, but processing them with the faculty member helps students to feel more comfortable the next time these issues arise.

During the clinical practicum, I encourage students to find new experiences to explore within the community. Students have the ability to revise or change some experiences after approval from me. For instance, a LPN to BSN pathway student with considerable experience working with terminally ill AIDS clients in a long-term setting asked to spend more time in the respite child playcare setting where he could get more experience with family assessment and caring for the children of AIDS-infected families. Students are encouraged to pursue clinical interests and address agency needs when appropriate. As a result of resignations, the AIDS respite child care program was short-staffed. When students were allowed to ride the van to pick up the children, something usually done by volunteers, it opened up a great opportunity for students to home visit and develop relationships with family members. One student said:

> There was no room for boredom, and the learning was continuous because the clinical had several rotation sites. I enjoyed the flexibility and the different places I was exposed to. We also had the choice of following up with any particular site or experience. I chose to follow a family I met through the respite child care program. The young mother had AIDS, but her 3-year-old boy was uninfected. I was able to do subsequent home visits with the child care coordinator and discuss the results of the child's Denver developmental exam with the parent. I learned a lot about this family's needs.

Student Supervision

Supervision of undergraduate nursing students in an HIV/AIDS community environment presents numerous challenges. These include developing sensitivity to this population group, limiting the number of students an agency can take at any given time, and availability of clients with HIV/AIDS. Therefore, in addition to direct supervision, I rely on feedback from preceptors and agency points of contact, and data from course requirements and activities such as student journals.

In addition to supervising students in the field, it is also my role to ensure the students are in a safe working environment, and that information is communicated and made accessible to them as things come up. I am a role model, influencing positive attitudes and practices in HIV/AIDS care.

It is not unusual for my 10 clinical students to be dispersed over 5 or 6 different locations involving several community agencies on any given day; 2 at a counseling and testing site, 3 at a substance abuse center, 1 at an infectious disease clinic with a nurse case manager, 1 at a high school for youth prevention counseling, and 2 to 3 at an AIDS respite child care center. I rely heavily on a beeper and my cellular phone to keep me accessible and in touch with my students in the community. Agency members are provided with a student schedule and my beeper number.

Course objectives are given to the agency and to the preceptors each semester. With the objectives, preceptors and agency contacts help to clarify the purpose of the experience and set the ground rules in their agencies. Guidelines for clinical faculty supervision are provided to all faculty and discussed prior to the beginning of the semester. Faculty supervision guidelines state that the faculty member must be present in at least one site or enroute to a site. Most clinical days, I find it possible to travel to three sites to supervise students. The use of preceptors or a strong contact person at each agency is essential. Experiences are often one-to-one learning that ensures close supervision of the student by the agency preceptor and facilitates accurate feedback to me. I seek out feedback about student performance and behavior from preceptors and agency contact persons on a weekly basis.

Course requirements and activities help to keep me abreast of student progress in the HIV/AIDS community experience. Students keep a journal of clinical activities for each clinical day. This activity not only provides a written record of students' critical thinking and application of scientific data to clinical practice, but also can be used as a part of the overall clinical evaluation. This activity is invaluable because it provides me with a record of the students' application of theory to clinical practice and evidence of critical thinking. I ask students to address cognitive, psychomotor, and affective domains in their journals. The cognitive domain allows students the opportunity to compare and contrast the clients' clinical picture and nursing diagnoses with textbooks, professional journals, and other literature. Students examine thoughts and feelings about the client and the clinical environment. From journal entries, I can also gauge the students' competence in collaborating with other health-care colleagues. Student clinical evaluation is based on the course objectives. I find this greatly facilitates supervision.

Box 10-2   Learning Exercise for Faculty Use

Plan a "brown bag" faculty development session. Invite two persons with HIV/AIDS and three health-care team members (for instance, a case manager, social worker, mental health volunteer) to be a part of a panel discussion concerning interdisciplinary counseling and social support of the HIV/AIDS client. Ask the following questions:

How do you define support? How do you define counseling?

What do you do well in these two areas?

How would you go about teaching student nurses to address the counseling and support needs of HIV/AIDS clients?

Summarize the discussion and use it to build consensus on the meaning of these terms, and the role of the faculty member and the student nurse on the interdisciplinary team.

Teaching Strategies to Promote Student Learning

Before I begin a discussion of strategies to promote student learning, it must be said that flexibility must be the guiding principle when designing teaching-learning strategies. I place a strong emphasis on experiential learning activities with critical reflection. These activities enable students to expand their consciousness and explore different ways of seeing HIV disease in their community (Canadian Nurses Association, 1996). One of the ways this is affected is through partnering students with clients with HIV disease, health professionals, and with members of community groups. Linked up with nursing students, individuals with HIV and AIDS, and their significant others can promote the students' comprehension of the realities of living with HIV disease. Students access these individuals initially by meeting them with the nurse case manager, mental health counselor, the child care coordinator or through other agency-based experiences. Persons with AIDS and their families are often enthusiastic to impart insights and knowledge they have gained through experience to ensure quality care for others experiencing HIV disease.

An essential strategy is the clinical conference. It is crucial to allow sharing of experiences and monitoring of student progress. In a community-based setting where students are scattered at different sites, coming together for conference is the glue that seals the experiences. Some conference time may be used for didactic teaching in HIV care in conjunction with the discussion of student learning experiences. Teaching-learning projects with clients are also excellent ways to facilitate student learning.

Placing students in collaborative roles with other staff is a very valuable strategy. The health team member need not be a nurse to be in a pivotal role in the coordination and delivery of HIV care. Therefore, nursing students can benefit greatly from a mentoring relationship with any member of the health-care team, but in particular, with the case manager. Case managers can be found just about anywhere HIV/AIDS care is delivered.

With the case manager mentor, students experience firsthand that consistency and trust in the relationship is created over a long period. Students spend several days with the nurse case manager as they attend to the day-to-day activities such as seeing clients and performing physical assessment. One junior nursing student's comments following her experiences with the nurse case manager serves as a helpful summary.

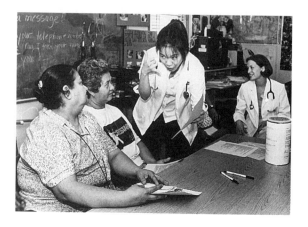

> *My experience began with the case manager, and this was a great way to begin. It's so nice to know that nurse clinicians still remember what it was like to be "green" and have empathy for our plight. The nurse case manager was wonderful about explaining everything she did and why. The client was wonderful about allowing me to "invade" his personal life. I learned a great deal about prophylaxsis, pathology, and human tragedy. "K" touched me deeply for many reasons. Although I held it together in his presence, I had to cry for awhile in solitude.*

This student's work with a dying client made this client's continuous decline and eventual death a reality for her. It helped the client's losses become more intimately known by the student nurse. The painful, yet beneficial, consequences of her encounter with this client deeply enriched the student's personal and professional life. She observed the nurse case manager intimately joining this client in his agonizing encounter with AIDS and helping him to emerge from one grief stage into another.

My faculty role in this experience, as with other student encounters with death and dying, is to encourage student instincts of humanity, that is, crying or feeling sad, and to support the student. I believe it is not only important for the faculty member to validate this experience for the student, but also facilitate use of self, agency staff, and the clinical group as mutual support systems. This provides an opportunity to share coping techniques, encourages person-to-person exchange based on identification and reciprocity, and may give the student access to a body of specialized information (Osterweis and colleagues 1984). In addition, students need to be exposed to different grief and bereavement frameworks with which to begin their own development of a workable grief model and their own personal style. Particularly congruent here is Shapiro's (1994) Family Development Model. In Shapiro's framework, grief is seen as a shared developmental process that involves a collaborative family identity in response to a new reality and a loss of a vital member (p 6). In a clinical environment, it is appropriate for faculty members to see agency staff and clinical groups as "family."

Perhaps nowhere else is that clinical "family" concept more apparent than in multidisciplinary team meetings where members support each other as they review care to clients. It is important for students to attend the agency multidisciplinary team meetings to view the case manager as the seam that connects all the other caregiver and services involved in the continuum of health-care delivery. It helps the student to appreciate that the multidisciplinary team approach to patients' needs and goals is tantamount in the client-provider relationship. Students learn that most pressing needs should be addressed first, and then interventions to maximize benefits can be taken. The faculty member may access this experience for students in a variety of settings: home care, hospitals, hospices, voluntary agencies, or managed care environments.

SCOPE OF FACULTY PRACTICE IN COMMUNITY-BASED HIV/AIDS SETTING

The paradigm shift in clinical nursing education has resulted in liberation and empowerment of both faculty and students. I see myself as the student's partner in just about every clinical venture. Flexibility is the rule, and students need not have similar learning experiences. The emphasis I place on experiential learning allows students to expand their conscientiousness, become critically reflective, and see the world through the clients' eyes. Caring pervades all we do.

My practice as nurse educator may at times include providing care for the clients as well as providing consultation or service on an agency committee or an advisory group. I take an active part in educating other health-care professionals at the clinical sites and also collaborate with students in their teaching projects. There is no better way to help a student see the melding together of theory and practice. In addition, students learn collaboration, and gain self-confidence from presenting with a professional.

In this chapter I have discussed my own experiences in the development and evolution of a clinical-based experience with an HIV/AIDS clinical placement. Through my own experience of establishing an HIV/AIDS community-based clinical, the greater the need or the perception of need for student services, the greater the likelihood of successful experiences at the agency. Likewise, an agency invested in teaching and training is more likely to support successful clinical experiences. The key to a successful alliance and partnership with the Juniper Program lies in having adequate time to solidify that relationship and responsiveness to the unique demands of the agency, the nursing students, and the clients.

Box 10-3 Learning Exercise for Faculty Use

Brainstorm all the social support services available to clients in your community who are living with HIV/AIDS. Create an easy-to-use resource list that includes name, address, phone number, e-mail address or Web site, and services.

References

Canadian Nurses Association (1996). Education for nurses: Practice issues and curriculum guidelines. Ottawa, Ontario: Canadian Nurses Association.

Norwood, SL (1998). Nurses as Consultants. Menlo Park, CA: Addison-Wesley.

Osterweis, M, et al. (1984). Bereavement reactions, consequences and care. Washington, DC: National Academy Press.

Shapiro, ER (1994). Grief as a family process. New York: Guildford Press.

CHAPTER 11

Teaching Students in a Home-care Setting

Susan W. Durham

Learning Objectives

1) Describe the faculty member's role and responsibilities in establishing an affiliation with a home-health agency.

2) Identify effective communication strategies to be used when interacting with interdisciplinary staff members in home health in relation to student issues.

3) Discuss the scope of nursing practice of undergraduate nursing students as it relates to other team members who work in home health.

4) Establish guidelines for an appropriate level of supervision for undergraduate nursing students placed in a home-health agency as their clinical site.

5) Discuss ways of creating effective learning experiences and developing teaching strategies used to aid students in applying their previously acquired nursing knowledge and skill in a home environment.

If nursing students are to be prepared to function in the present health-care environment, then they must be permitted to gain experience in settings that have not traditionally been used as clinical placements. Nurse educators should be prepared to embrace the realities of a health-care system where nursing care is performed in community-based settings so that they prepare their students to meet the changing health-care needs (Oesterle & O'Callaghan 1996). Whether you are currently involved in a community-based nursing program or are just using selective community placements to meet the needs of your curriculum, this chapter will assist you in better preparing your students to function in the home-care environment. It will detail ways that a home-health agency and a nursing program can form a partnership that benefits both while providing a legitimate place to accomplish course objectives and perform the skills that students need for clinical practice.

FACULTY, STUDENT, AND STAFF ROLES AND RESPONSIBILITIES IN A HOME-HEALTH CLINICAL

Until recently home-health agencies have been used primarily for community health clinical placements for undergraduate nursing students. The use of a home-health agency as an alternative site for our senior, medical/surgical preceptorship seemed like a logical way to offer students a setting that would acknowledge the shift in the delivery of nursing care from the hospital to the home. The benefits of such an affiliation were very clear to our college and were in keeping with our recent curriculum change to a community-based focus. Discussions began with a large home-health agency in our area to investigate the possibility of an agreement for a clinical placement. We proposed something similar to the Bolton Model out of Case Western Reserve where senior nursing students are partnered with a registered nurse with a BSN degree for a concentrated clinical experience. In this model the preceptor functions in the role of clinical instructor, and the faculty member provides intensive guidance and supervision to the preceptor and the student through weekly joint conferences. The faculty member is immediately available by phone or beeper 24 hours a day, 7 days a week while the students are in this clinical. The student works the preceptor's schedule for a specified number of weeks. According to Loughman, "Clear student practice guidelines and close student supervision by the faculty and the preceptor dictate the experience" (1997 p 193). The faculty member may make evaluation home visits with the student when necessary. Table 11–1 summarizes roles for each position.

The home-health agency agreed to take 5 senior students for a 7-week clinical experience where the students would work with the preceptors' schedule for approximately 32 hours per week. As part of the agreement, we negotiated things like scope of practice, student skill level and autonomy, and clinical competence. The next big hurdle was to find home-health nurses who would be willing to make the commitment to precept students.

The home-health association was able to see the advantages that such an affiliation would bring to its agency. "Educational programs can offer considerable benefits to enhance the overall clinical practice of a home care agency" (Loughman 1997 p 190). Some of the benefits include supporting continuing education, assisting with research and publication, and sharing educational resources. Other possible advantages are reduced orientation efforts and costs, increased referrals and a view of potential recruits for hire (Loughman 1997). All of these positive aspects can be very appealing to administrators, but the home-health nurses are the real key to the success of the affiliation because the burden of precepting is on them (Yoder et al. 1997). They must clearly see the advantage that this effort brings to their daily practice. An excerpt of my experience in beginning an affiliation with a home-health agency for our senior precepted clinical follows. As we were preparing for the clinical, the things that the preceptors were concerned about and the things that I thought were important were very different.

Setting the Stage

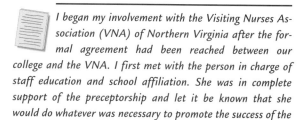

I began my involvement with the Visiting Nurses Association (VNA) of Northern Virginia after the formal agreement had been reached between our college and the VNA. I first met with the person in charge of staff education and school affiliation. She was in complete support of the preceptorship and let it be known that she would do whatever was necessary to promote the success of the

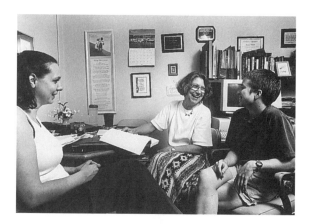

Table 11-1

Faculty, Student, and Staff Roles

NURSE PRECEPTOR	BSN STUDENT	FACULTY MEMBER	AGENCY MENTOR
Serves as the student's clinical mentor.	Formulates personal objectives for the clinical experience based on course objectives.	Coordinates the various aspects of the course including implementation and evaluation.	Coordinates the implementation of the student's clinical experience.
Collaborates with the faculty member.	Establishes a professional relationship with the preceptor.	Participates in the clinical supervision of the nursing students.	Provides on-call consultation on a 24-hour basis while students are affiliated with agency.
Works with the student in planning, organizing, and providing care to a small group of patients.	Follows agency polices and procedures.	Provides on-call consultation to student, preceptor, and agency on a 24-hour basis during the course.	
Provides feedback to the student on his/her progress on a daily basis.	Becomes autonomous within the role of student nurse and within agency parameters.	Functions as a liaison between the agency and university.	
Assists the student in becoming autonomous within the student role.	Communicates any problems or potential problems to preceptor or faculty member.	Assumes overall responsibility for all aspects of the course.	
In collaboration with the faculty member, evaluates student performance.	Participates in the evaluation sessions with the preceptor and faculty member.	Evaluates the agency at the end of the experience.	

affiliation. She and I spoke about possible preceptor candidates, about students' scope of practice, faculty roles and responsibilities, clinical performance supervision, and agency policy. We decided that she would first meet on her own with the prospective preceptors to promote a free and open forum. Then I met with those nurses who were truly interested, presented the course overview, and answered questions regarding the scope of the course.

The educational coordinator and I agreed to let the nurses lead the first meeting with their questions. They were a difficult audience. Many nurses seemed suspicious that they were not getting the full story. Their concerns revolved around issues that I thought were insignificant but to them were very important. One item that disturbed them the most was having the students ride in their car from the agency to the client's house. It seemed an intrusion into their personal space, like giving someone the use of their office. I thought they would be worried about such things as scope of practice and clinical supervision, but they were concentrating much more on a personal level. A few days into the preceptorship, the issues discussed during the first meeting eventually became nonissues. Many nurses found that they loved having the students on visits and in their car between visits. It gave them the opportunity to collaborate and brief the students on the next client. Precepting was a new concept for them and took some adjustment time.

The benefits of precepting need to be articulated very clearly to the home-health nurses in your first meeting, as does a sincere acknowledgment of their concerns. According to Loughman (1997), the benefits of precepting include

- the student's ability to offer the preceptor a fresh view of a situation
- the student's ability to identify new and developing symptoms in their clients
- the student's ability to reinforce and share the responsibilities of patient teaching
- the opportunity for preceptors to give back to their profession
- the opportunity for preceptors to look at their self-practice to incorporate new ideas

The following is an example of how one of my students was able to offer a fresh perspective in solving a problem with a home-care client and of the preceptor's openness in letting that happen.

A FRESH LOOK AT A LONG-TERM PROBLEM

This student began visiting a long-term client who was struggling with a way to sort out her medication schedule. The client was on many medications and was also illiterate so she was not able to read the directions on the bottles. The nurse had tried several methods to assist her in remembering her schedule, none of which seemed to be working. The student began to work with this client and was aware of the problem. She came up with an idea to color-code all of the medications and use symbols for the time of day that the medications were to be taken. She glued a sample of each pill onto a small poster board and drew a symbol next to the pill representing the time of day that the pill was to be taken (for instance, half sun for morning and full sun for noon, dark circle for bedtime, and so forth). With the permission of the preceptor she called the doctor to see if brands of pills could be found that could make each pill a different color. They were able to work it out and the client, for the first time, was able to understand when to take each medication. Her condition improved markedly.

Because of a little creativity and the willingness of the preceptor to accept a new idea from a student, a client became compliant with her medications and a problem was solved. The nurse was very grateful to the student. "Nurses can find new energy and enthusiasm

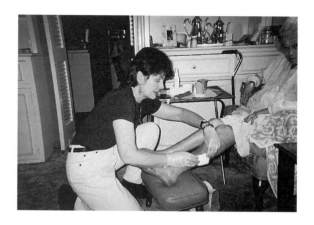

when viewing home care through students' eyes" (Loughman 1997, p 190). Just recently one of two preceptors who were job sharing said to me, "Our student is brighter than Joan and me together, but it is not a threatening thing. She stimulates us by asking complicated questions that motivate us to study our 'patho' as we share with her the finer points of home-care nursing." These preceptors and their student developed a model collaborative relationship built on mutual respect and admiration.

The barriers to the success of an affiliation can be very different from what might be assumed. The problems of scope of practice, student autonomy, and clinical competence are the issues many agencies wrestle with when accepting student nurses into their midst. However, the nursing administrator's view of a situation may be very different from that of the home-health-nursing staff. This happened in our affiliation during the first semester that our students were placed in home health. Because of our inexperience in dealing with home-health issues, a problem arose that neither our college nor the agency administration anticipated.

AT A PERSONAL LEVEL

The first semester at the home-health agency seemed to go really well. I had met with each preceptor at least once a week to discuss student progress and to address any problems. The students were hand-chosen so they all had strong clinical skills. The preceptors seemed to enjoy working with them, and the feedback had all been positive.

During my weekly meetings with the preceptors, I had a list of questions that I asked centering on the issues of scope of practice, student autonomy, clinical performance, and so on. There were very few complaints and a minimal number of problems. I was feeling really positive about the experience and had visions of a long collaborative relationship with the VNA, with nurses lining up to precept the next semester.

The educational coordinator at the VNA suggested that we have an end-of-semester meeting to thank the preceptors and to discuss any areas for improvement. The director of my undergraduate program decided to come to the meeting, and I told her that the meeting should be uneventful. Well, I could not have been more wrong. After the initial discussion about the joys of the student-preceptor relationships, there was an angry explosion from the nurses who were compensated on a per-diem basis. They were livid. The agency had told them that it supported education, but what no one thought of was their loss in productivity and income during the preceptorship. All of the salaried nurses were paid their usual salary in spite of a drop in productivity, but the per-diem nurses did not get reimbursed for student visits. About half of our original preceptors were paid per diem. Many of these nurses were dropping their students off at the end of the day and then going on to do additional visits to maintain their income. Not one of the nurses ever mentioned that to me during our meetings and I did not know enough to ask such questions. The emotion and anger expressed in the meeting was totally unexpected by everyone. The administrators at the agency were just as surprised as I was, and I was totally embarrassed that I did not warn my director of undergraduate programs about the problem. I left the meeting in tears.

The Medicare Coverage of Services, Transmittal Revision 222, allows for students to make independent visits that are also billable for Medicare if they meet a very specific set of guidelines (Humphrey & Milone-Nuzzo 1996). In many instances Medicaid and some third-party payers have followed suit. In our situation, the home-health agency immediately said that it would arrange to reimburse per-diem nurses for student visits. These nurses also realized that, although their productivity dropped in the early part of preceptorship, it nearly doubled after students began making independent visits. I learned that clinical questions were not the only important things to discuss with the preceptors during our meetings but a sensitivity and openness to the personal issues affecting precepting were just as important.

Communication

Effective communication with the preceptors and students is one of your most important roles as a faculty member involved in a home-care affiliation. In home health it is more challenging to stay in touch with the preceptors than in a hospital setting because of the geographical obstacles inherent in this specialty. When a student is precepted in a hospital, arriving at the hospital on a day when a preceptor and student are scheduled to work, guarantees the faculty member an opportunity to see the preceptor. When students are making home visits, they are not in the agency except at the beginning of the day when planning visits, or at the end of the day when finishing up. Because of the wide visiting area and its lack of proximity to many agency offices, not all preceptors go into the office every day. Sometimes students must drive to the preceptor's home and begin their visits from there. What I have found works best is to choose specific days and times each week to be available in the agency office for consultation. I usually ask the preceptors which hours of the day and days of the week are most convenient. Then I find a central location in the agency office and bring work or reading to keep me occupied while I wait. The preceptors know where I am, and they generally check in with me when they arrive. They then fit our meeting in around their end-of-day phone calls and charting. The students do the same thing. At the beginning of the semester during our weekly meetings, I meet with the students and preceptors separately. Relationship building is still going on, and sometimes it is necessary to help the student or the preceptor work through personality differences or communication problems with each other. Early on, they feel more comfortable speaking honestly and freely without the other present. As the weeks go by, when things are clearly going well, I generally meet with the student and the preceptor jointly. After the collaborative relationship has developed and solidified, feedback flows more freely from one to the other.

An attempt is made at the beginning of the semester to match student traits with those of the preceptor to promote a more cohesive relationship. This works well once the affiliation is established and the faculty member is familiar with the personalities of the home-health nurses. When an association is new and the faculty member and the preceptors do not know each other very well, it is much more difficult to pair preceptors with compatible students. If the faculty member is not acquainted with the nurses being considered for preceptorship, the educational coordinator can give input to the faculty member regarding the personality traits of the home-health nurses. Generally students have the same preceptor throughout the entire clinical rotation. If two nurses job-share, then the student is assigned to both nurses but never more than that. Students frequently go on visits with other nurses for a day to gain a new experience or to meet an interesting patient, but they are accountable to their nurse at all times. This relationship gives the experience continuity and gives the student consistency. When it is time to evaluate student performance, the faculty member can count on the preceptor being totally familiar with the student's performance and being able to offer specific examples of how the student is meeting or not meeting the course objectives.

During our second semester at the VNA, we had an incident where a student and a preceptor could not have been more of a mismatch. It was almost a disaster.

Wrong for Each Other

I have the student's complete biographical data sheets prior to the beginning of the clinical because I do not always know them or their clinical preferences. Some of the information that is requested is work experience, education, personal interests, and professional goals. I also ask their age and for three words that best describe them. Before I knew the VNA staff that well, I compiled the student biographical data and gave that information to the VNA's educational coordinator, and she made the assignments. In this particular case, she made a logical choice based on the information that she was given.

She paired a student who had been an experienced LPN with a preceptor who had also been a LPN and seemed to have similar interests. The preceptor happened to be a vegetarian, and the student was not. Not only was she not a vegetarian, she seemed completely oblivious to the fact that eating a large cheese steak submarine sandwich in her preceptor's car was inappropriate. The situation went from bad to worse. The student's insensitivity to the preceptor's preferences and personal space began to tinge everything that the student did in the preceptor's eyes. This preceptor was quiet and self-contained. The student was aggressive and flamboyant. They could not have been a worse match. By the time the preceptor confided in me that she had a personality conflict with the student, we were too far into the semester to change the preceptor assignment. I had several conferences with the student about sensitivity, and she really had a difficult time understanding the problem. I did a lot of creative things like placing the student with nurse specialists, supervising her visits myself, and sending her out with other disciplines. When the student began making independent home visits, things improved, but we all barely survived the semester. Getting to know the nursing staff a little better over time has helped avoid such diverse match-ups.

Flexibility

Faculty flexibility is the second most important role in supporting a home-health nurse involved in a preceptor experience. Schedule changes are inevitable because of client problems or other uncontrollable events. Home-health nurses are under a great deal of stress, and it is really damaging to the faculty-preceptor relationship to make the preceptor feel bad about missing or changing a meeting appointment. Sometimes this means smiling in spite of my own frustration after waiting for an hour or so for a preceptor just to find out that she is stuck in traffic or has had a problem with her client and must cancel on me. Most of the preceptors have cellular phones, so they are very considerate about calling or paging me immediately when they know they have a problem. Once in awhile, it is necessary to have the weekly preceptor conference by phone. I never do that more than once or twice a semester, but sometimes it is unavoidable. So we talk at night after things have settled down in the preceptor's day. At times I meet preceptors and students near a client's home or for lunch in their visiting area. I try to be as flexible as I can be because I know that the home-health nurses' schedule is driven by so many variables out of their control.

Some of the preceptors use e-mail to communicate nonurgent messages to me regarding such things as student progress, alternative experiences, or schedule changes. Voice mail is also used extensively in home health. The nurses access their voice mail several times a day. If a nonurgent message needs to be communicated to preceptors, I leave a message on their voice mail and then page them to the voice mail number for a call back. When they see their voice mail number on their pager, they know to access their voice mail before going on to the next visit. That way they get the message fairly soon, yet the continuity of the visit is not interrupted by a phone call. Immediate messages are communicated via pagers or beepers and answered quickly by the preceptor. Modern technology has made it fairly easy to stay in touch with the home-health nurse in spite of the geographical obstacles.

DEVELOPING LEARNING EXPERIENCES THROUGH EFFECTIVE TEACHING STRATEGIES

The focus of the clinical experience is to assist students in meeting the course objectives in a home-health environment. To do this we feel that the students need to be aware of the unique properties involved in delivering care in the home. Some of the things that I address with the students at the beginning and throughout the semester include

- historical perspective regarding the role of the home-health nurse
- appreciation for a more multidisciplinary approach to nursing care
- awareness of the unique aspects of infection control in an environment with varying degrees of cleanliness
- respect for the issues of personal safety and client safety in situations where the environment is out of provider control
- documentation needed for the purposes of reimbursement of Medicare, Medicaid, and Managed Care
- client and family education in the home
- medication management in the home
- evaluation of unlicensed assistive personnel (UAPs) in the role of Home Health Aid (HHA)
- referrals for community and medical resources (Glavinspiehs & Gajdalo 1997)

Some of the ways in which students absorb all of this information is through laboratory simulations, journal writing, case study analysis, clinical conferencing, and through student partnerships.

Laboratory Simulations

In preparing for other clinical experiences, our college has used the nursing technology laboratory to assist students in fine-tuning their clinical skills before having to perform them in a real-life situation. The nursing technology lab can be used in a similar way to prepare students to function in a home environment. Oermann & Gaberson (1998) states, "Simulations allow learners to experience a situation and gain an awareness of their feelings, perceptions, and responses before facing or encountering the situation in a clinical setting" (1998, p 189). Prior to the first home visit, students in the lab are encouraged to think about some of the situations they might encounter in the home. One way of doing this is by setting up a section of your nursing technology lab to look like a client's home. A regular bed can be used with pieces of furniture that might be found in the home. Then your faculty can write scenarios that stimulate student thought regarding the kinds of challenges that may be encountered. Box 11–1 is an example of a scenario that could be used to stimulate students to think critically when walking into the client's environment for the first time.

This scenario includes the use of assessment and clinical judgment, phone contact with another provider, communicating the purpose of a visit to the client, considerations regarding proper bag technique, the possibility of resource referral, the performance of client teaching, and documentation. Role-playing this scenario will encourage the student to think about the many variables involved with giving nursing care in the home. Some of the challenges presented make it difficult to accomplish the objectives of the visit. You can design your scenarios to help students think through complicated situations in preparation for the unknowns that home health has to offer.

| Box 11-1 | Learning Exercise for Faculty Use |

Critical Thinking Scenario

You are visiting a client, Ms. R, who has Type II diabetes and is being visited for the purpose of nutritional education and diabetic teaching regarding self-monitoring of blood glucose and self-administration of insulin. The client is 65 years old and is a widow who lives with her 38-year-old daughter, her 16-year-old granddaughter, and her granddaughter's 2-month-old baby boy. Both her daughter and granddaughter are unmarried and on Medicaid. They live in a single-family home that is in a state of disrepair. As you approach the house, you notice broken and missing boards on the porch where the paint is badly peeling and in some instances nonexistent. You enter the home through the living room, which is large and furnished with upholstered furniture that is torn and soiled.

You state the purpose of your visit, and ask if you can get started. The client is very upset about her great-grand baby. She asks you to take a look at the baby because she is concerned about a few recent episodes of diarrhea. She and her daughter usher you into a downstairs bedroom just off of the living-room area. The baby is lying naked on a bare, dirty mattress that was recently soiled with watery, greenish-yellow stool. You look for a place to put your bag, and decide to hang it on the doorknob. There is a box of Pampers on the bed so you wash your hands, put on your gloves, clean off the baby's bottom, and pull a Pamper from the box for the purpose of applying it. As you pull the Pamper from the box, a cockroach falls from the clean diaper onto the baby's face and crawls across his head. You are the only one who jumps. You inquire about the baby's diet and discover that they had fed him Gerber's cherry cobbler last evening. Just then the baby's mother comes downstairs on her way to see some friends. When introduced to you, she makes no eye contact and gives no acknowledgment of your presence. She leaves without even glancing at the baby. The baby's grandmother begins screaming at her daughter and goes on about how her daughter should have never kept this baby. You ask if they have a baby doctor, and the grandmother says that they take him to the neighborhood clinic. After putting on the diaper and assessing the baby's hydration status, you call the clinic for the grandmother. The instructions are to stop all food and give the baby formula diluted to 50% strength with boiled water. Full-strength formula should not be resumed until the diarrhea stops. You instruct her to count the number of stools and the frequency and amount of the wet diapers because they can give her an indication of dehydration. You tell her to call the clinic doctor if the baby continues to have the loose stool and if he develops a fever.

You ask Ms. R if she would mind talking for awhile about her diabetes. She suggests going into the living room. There are no hard-backed chairs. So you start out by standing while you talk. Ms. R insists that you have a seat. You sit near her on the sofa because you have to do her finger stick. As you are discussing her 24-hour diet recall, you feel a dampness soaking through your skirt to your skin. You realize that your skirt is completely wet. You decide to hold your bag so that you do not have to place it on the floor because you have seen a few more roaches climbing on walls. You can hardly keep your mind on your teaching, wondering what you are sitting in. Ms. R demonstrates the finger stick to you, and another nurse has filled the insulin syringes for the week so you remove one from the refrigerator and give the injection. You will return tomorrow to teach the client injection technique. You make sure the client knows how to check her blood sugar before her evening insulin, and that she knows what to do if she develops the signs and symptoms of hypoglycemia. You rapidly say goodbye. Your visit has gone 30 minutes over your estimated time. Fortunately, you live about 20 minutes away from there, so you can go home and take a quick shower and change your clothes before returning to the office. Ms. R was your last client for the day.

Make a list of things that were infection-control issues in this home.

At any time during your visit was infection control compromised?

At what point did you put yourself at risk during the visit and what could have been done to prevent it?

Should you have gotten involved in the care of the infant and why?

> **Box 11-1** Learning Exercise for Faculty Use—cont'd
>
> Based on the family dynamics, are there any referrals that could be made that would help the family with its problems?
>
> How does using role-play in this situation help you to better prepare for future, unexpected circumstances in the home?

Journals

Clinical journals can be a valuable tool in providing students with an opportunity to document their responses to clinical experiences. Journals are also a way of expressing feelings and engaging in dialogue with teachers about them (Oermann & Gaberson 1998). They also offer a means of evaluating the critical-thinking abilities of students throughout a clinical course (Callister 1993). They are especially valuable in a precepted clinical because the instructor is not directly observing the student's performance. The journal, therefore, provides the instructor with a window into the clinical experience. In our clinical preceptorship, students are required to submit weekly clinical journals, which are evaluated according to the following criteria:

- Perceptiveness in identifying personal objectives and learning needs
- Thoroughness in recording and responding to clinical experiences
- Objectivity and insight into their own performance
- Thoroughness in assessing and analyzing decision-making abilities
- Consistency of entries

The faculty give feedback on journal entries in an attempt to encourage pertinent client follow-up, to stimulate analytic thought regarding nursing actions, and to validate emotional responses to student experiences (Glavinspiehs & Gajdalo 1997). If journals are in notebook form, feedback is given weekly with a week delay from collection to distribution. Some faculty encourage the use of e-mail entries. The value of this format is that it provides the student with almost immediate feedback from the faculty member.

Some of the emotional responses that my home-care students have written about are the culture shock in observing different value systems, the distractions present in the home environment, the unpredictable situations and dynamics among family members, the dichotomy in the state and conditions of the homes, the scarcity of supplies, the autonomy of the home-health nurse, the importance of the nurse-patient relationship, the power of the human spirit in the home-bound ill, and the daily frustrations in dealing with managed care. Our course uses the journal as a graded component of the final clinical grade. This works very well in our course; however, some schools use journals as a nongraded component of a clinical experience.

Case Study Analysis

During a clinical preceptorship, the faculty member has very little opportunity to observe the direct care performed by their students in a clinical setting. The feedback from the preceptor, the descriptions of student performances, and student self-evaluation are some of the means used by faculty to formulate an accurate summative evaluation to produce a final course grade. Our faculty feels the need for multiple sources of data to make accurate judgments about the quality of a student's clinical performance. Oermann & Gaberson suggest that writing assignments provide effective strategies for evaluating a student's problem solving, decision making, and critical-thinking skills (1998). We decided to use a case study requirement as a basis for the evaluation of a student's ability to do a comprehensive analysis of a client's problems and to provide evidence upon which her or his clinical decisions have been based. The case study is another component of the final clinical grade. The students in home care include in their assessment the many challenges and barriers that impact the recovery process of the homebound client.

Clinical Conferences

Because home health is in such a solitary practice setting, there is not as much opportunity for students to interact with each other in the clinical context. It is not like the hospital where they can go out into the hallway and bring another student into the client's room to listen to an interesting heart sound or to see an unusual rash pattern. I felt strongly that we had to find ways to bring our home-care students together to share and discuss their experiences. Even though students were working many different schedules and were spread out over a large geographical area, I decided it was still important for us to come together as a group to discuss and process the events of the week. Because the students were already scheduled for a 2-hour per week seminar course, I added another hour of clinical conference time to that class period for clinical sharing. That worked well for us. During our clinical conferences, students eagerly shared the events and experiences of the week. They anxiously awaited updates on other students' clients to find out how a particular situation was resolved. It is clear that the home-care experience has made an indelible impact on their view of their clients. They feel that they will no longer make assumptions about why clients are noncompliant with discharge instructions or medication regimens. They forever will consider caregiver support, environmental issues and hazards, insurance benefits, and client access to transportation and treatment resources in doing their discharge planning. In these conferences students are able to share resources for patient education and continuing education. They offer each other emotional support in handling difficult client situations, and they laugh and cry together. In the following description of a difficult situation, a student shared his frustrations regarding the injustices shown to his client in a managed care situation.

VENTING FRUSTRATIONS

During one clinical conference, a student shared the events of a particularly frustrating week and his disillusionment with the managed care system. He was caring for a client who had been newly diagnosed with AIDS. She was in the very late stages when she finally sought medical treatment. She had been hospitalized for a few days where she was started on the Protease cocktail and then was discharged. The managed care agency had only approved two visits for follow-up and teaching. The home-health nurse was tasked with doing her admission, which takes at least 2 hours and then beginning the teaching about her medication regimen. This woman was so ill and weak that she could barely concentrate. Two visits were not enough, but that was what they had to work with.

The student and the nurse went on the first visit and, working together, they were able to get through the admission assessment and paperwork and just begin the instruction on the medications. The client was so worn out that she could not absorb any more information. Both the student and the nurse decided that it would be better to let the client rest and begin the next day on the remainder of the teaching. They were also feeling that two visits were not going to be enough. When they returned to the agency at the end of the visit, there was a message from this client's managed care insurance to say they withdrew the approval for the second visit. The home-health nurse had to call and beg the managed care company for the second visit and update them on the client's condition. The company really resisted, and the nurse in frustration told them that they need not worry about extended care for this client because she was going to be dead soon and then they would be happy. She did finally get the second visit approved, but when she arrived in the office the next morning, she received a message that the client had been rushed to the hospital's intensive care unit during the night. The nurse was so frustrated because she felt that the client should have never been discharged from the hospital in the first place. The student had a huge dose of "reality shock." He shared his frustration with his fellow students, and everyone tried to support him in his despair and frustration.

This particular experience monopolized the entire conference but was a great learning time for students. We discussed ways that nursing as a profession could effect change to prevent situations such as this and ways the nurse and student can become effective advocates for clients who are treated unfairly.

Student Partnerships

I have always encouraged student partnering when doing home visits if there are appropriate opportunities to do so. Some of the reasons why I encourage joint home visiting are so a student is given the opportunity to perform a skill not yet performed, to observe an interesting patient on someone else's caseload, to offer support or assistance if the preceptor cannot be there when a second pair of hands are needed, to encourage camaraderie, and to decrease anxiety levels when a little moral support is needed. The clients love the extra attention that students are able to give them, so they are generally receptive to student visits. Sometimes students collaborate and trade preceptors for the day. It is good for them to have the opportunity to observe another nurse's style of nursing care and gain an experience that their particular caseload does not offer at that time.

Working with Other Disciplines

One advantage of placing nursing students in a home-health-care setting is the opportunity to interface with providers from other disciplines. Home-health nurses function in a true collaborative role in the care of their clients. Many agencies employ a staff of social workers, physical and occupational therapists, and home-health aids who are all a part of a team approach to the client's recovery. When placed in a home-health agency for a clinical experience, nursing students are given daily opportunities to collaborate with these other disciplines as they perform their nursing care. They may do a joint visit with a physical therapist and learn a new way of assisting a client in accomplishing activities of daily living. A joint visit with a social worker can offer a student insight into problems arising from family dynamics. Meeting in the home with the HHA can give a student the opportunity to learn the client's routine, offer the chance to teach the HHA the reasoning behind a particular treatment regimen, or accomplish a periodic quality of care evaluation. These interdisciplinary interactions broaden students' scope of nursing practice and teach them the importance of the collaborative nature of the health professions.

Jobs for new nursing graduates are not yet available in home health immediately upon graduation. However, home health is still a valuable clinical placement for undergraduate nursing students. As the number of hospital beds has decreased, the acute-care settings are not able to support all of the clinical sites needed by nursing programs. Therefore, it is necessary to seek out clinical placements beyond the acute-care setting. A partnership with a home-health agency can offer valid and worthwhile learning experiences for nursing students. This new venue supports a shift in the philosophical basis for student placements. In a community-based curriculum, instead of looking at clinical settings in the context of programmatic needs, student placements are based more on the community's needs and ways the curriculum can support them. Regardless of the extent to which your program has shifted to a community-based approach to nursing education, home health can offer valuable opportunities for your students to learn and develop into competent practitioners.

References

Callister, LC (1993). The use of student journals in nursing education: Making meaning out of clinical experience. J Nurs Educ 32, 185–186.

Glavinspiehs, C & Gajdalo, J (1997). A meaningful clinical experience in home healthcare for associate degree graduate nurses. Nurs Educ 22(2), 33–37.

Humphrey, C & Milone-Nuzzo, P (1996). Medicare Coverage of Services (Transmittal Revision 222). Orientation to Home Care Nursing. Gaithersburg, MD: Aspen.

Loughman, KA (1997). The essentials for managing student home healthcare experiences. Home Healthc Nurs 15(3), 189–196.

Oermann, MH & Gaberson, KB (1998). Evaluation and testing in nursing education. New York: Springer.

Oesterle, M & O'Callaghan, D (1996). The changing health care environment: Impact on curriculum and faculty. N&HI: Perspectives on Community, 17(2) 78–81.

Yoder, MK, et al. (1997.) Agency-university collaboration: Home care early in the student curriculum. Home Healthc Nurs 15(7), 493–499.

CHAPTER 12
Teaching Students in a Faith Community

Margaret M. Moss

"Formal education is the beginning of the process of lifelong learning."—Thomas Jefferson, 1825 (Baron 1993)

Learning Objectives

1) Describe the history of nursing in a faith community.
2) Identify the steps involved in establishing a community-based clinical in a faith community.
3) Ascertain appropriate learning experiences for students in a faith community.
4) Discuss the importance of maintaining safety for students and clients in a faith community.
5) Describe teaching strategies to promote student learning.

A student offers her perspective on differences between community-based and hospital nursing:

My observations and, more often, my experiences gave me an appreciation for the differences between community-based and hospital nursing. Often these differences made themselves inconveniently known during a home visit. The following are some of the differences I uncovered at my faith community clinical site:

In a hospital...If I don't know the answer to a patient's particular question, I can sneak around the corner, look it up, and return with an answer better than I could ever have come up with on my own.

If I forgot to bring it (whatever it is) with me, I can walk down the hall and get it, or at least borrow someone else's.

It is never so quiet that a patient can hear my stomach growl during a therapeutic silence.

I know which door is the bathroom, and which is the closet!

I rarely have to worry about stepping on the patient's pet cat, and a dog doesn't attempt to identify me with his nose as I get in the door.

I don't have to worry that the patient may offer me a slice of steaming, tempting, delicious hospital food.

Patient teaching is never interrupted by the noise of the neighbor yelling at his dog to "shut up and stop barking."

SOB is not an insult, "void" has nothing to do with what you did to a check you wrote for the wrong amount, and BM is not a brand of baked beans.

I know there are many more differences, but I don't want to spoil any more surprises. A week in a community-based setting can create a list twice as long. On a more serious note, despite the many differences between community-based and hospital nursing, the goal is the same... patient care. This means caring enough to look up what you don't know, to share what you do know, and to never let the final answer to a patient's question be, " I don't know."

The decade of the 1990s experienced dramatic changes in the health-care delivery system. Development of innovative models of community-based health care is mandatory to address the myriad of changes facing the current health-care delivery system. New models must focus on health promotion and disease prevention and emphasize individual responsibilities and self-care. As evidenced throughout this textbook, community-based clinical sites are the essence of practice for our nursing students. Community-based experiences for students foster learning about people within the context of home and community and offer the best promise for students to learn the complex human dynamics of real life and develop a holistic perspective required for independent nursing practice (Clark & Cody 1994). One innovative model is that of parish nursing. Parish nursing is one of the newer, yet older, models of health-care delivery. The history of nursing is replete with examples of religious orders or congregations providing care for the sick. Churches have been involved in the delivery of health care for more than 2000 years (Weis et al. 1997).

Parish nursing is defined as the practice of "holistic health care" within a faith community, emphasizing the relationship between faith and health (Bergquist & King 1994, Biddix & Brown 1999). Faith community in this chapter refers to any gathering place where there is an assembly of people whose beliefs about God combine with a common identity, a shared history, a regular worship and common values (Solari-Twadell & McDermott 1999). The revival of the modern concept of faith-community-based health ministry occurred in 1984 and is credited to Rev. Granger Westberg, a retired Lutheran minister and hospital chaplain. He believed that faith communities could play a larger role in health promotion and disease prevention and that nurses had the special gifts to implement this practice. Westberg approached Lutheran General Hospital (LGH), a 608-bed hospital located in Park Ridge, Illinois, regarding partnering with a parish nurse program. LGH had long been a leader in pastoral care for its patients, and it showed immediate interest in the idea of partnering with local congregations in a parish nurse project. An administrative team from LGH was organized to plan and implement the first institutionally based program. Six congregations were willing to participate and agreed to a 3-year trial period. In 1985 the first parish nurse network was established with six parish nurses. This initial project was immediately successful, and it became apparent that these six nurses had made extensive inroads into assisting people, many in the early stages of illness, by their presence in the faith community. The faith community is a natural support system that enables access to all age, ethnic, and faith groups, in urban and rural sites, and from all socioeconomic levels. Faith communities have emerged as the one organization in our society most suited for leadership in the field of health promotion and disease prevention. In 1998 there were an estimated 3,000 nurses in faith communities serving in rural, urban, suburban, and inner-city settings throughout the country. Granger Westberg died in February 1999, and he will be remembered as the Father of the Parish Nurse Concept. His vision became reality.

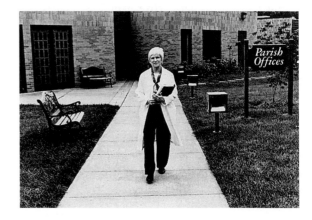

DEVELOPMENT OF A PARTNERSHIP FOR HEALTH

In the fall of 1996, I was asked to do a spring community-based clinical with 10 junior nursing students. I had a choice between assuming an existing clinical on the George Mason University (GMU) campus or establishing a new clinical site at a church. The development of this parish clinical was initiated by a faculty member who was also a respected member of this parish community. She and the associate dean of GMU's College of Nursing and Health Science met several times with the pastor to define and describe the kinds of services that the nursing students and faculty could provide to the faith community, services that were within the capabilities of the students and that would meet the course objectives.

GMU's College of Nursing and Health Science adapted a parish nursing model to deliver holistic health care in a faith community. In this model, students are not involved in doing parish nursing as defined in the literature (Solari-Twadell & McDermott 1999), but they do address the physiological, sociological, and psychological perspectives of health and healing in their work with clients. They refer all major spiritual matters to the faith community pastor, priest, or pastoral ministers. GMU developed a partnership for HEALTH with The Church of the Nativity (referred to as Nativity) in January, 1997. The purpose of the partnership is to promote holistic health to the faith community and to prevent disease while facilitating the education of nursing students. The acronym HEALTH was selected to denote Health counselor, Educator, Advocator, Liaison to the community, Teacher and Health promoter. This was the foundation for the Nativity/GMU Partnership for HEALTH. The pastor was identified as the contact person for the faculty and students.

With a sense of adventure in my soul, I chose Nativity as my clinical site. I immediately sought out another faculty member, Dr. Dawn Rigney, whom I knew had experience in parish nursing. She recommended I read *Parish Nursing: The Developing Practice,* edited by Solari-Twadell and colleagues (1990), and she also suggested activities she and her students had planned, implemented, and evaluated in their church site. In addition, I spoke with a nursing colleague who had experience working with a parish nurse. These collaborative efforts proved to be extremely important and helpful in the preliminary stages of development of the Nativity clinical.

As I began to gather information, I formulated limitless ideas and possibilities for student experiences at this new clinical site. (What are some of the ideas going through your mind as you read this? Jot them down on a sheet of paper!) On a cold, windy day in early January I took a drive out to the new clinical site, and as I drove around the neighborhood, I noticed many large, lovely homes, yet many areas of townhouses, low-income housing, and lots of shopping centers, a regional library, some fast food restaurants, and no hospital or emergency care facility for at least 15 miles. While on this drive, I made a stop at the church. Nativity is a very large, simple, and peaceful place where I experienced good vibrations that my students and I could make an impact on this faith community.

As I drove back to the university, I reflected upon the fact that this faith community has a membership of 4,000 families from which to draw potential clients and a list of homebound individuals. The attached school has 250 children in grades kindergarten through eight and a variety of activities including a before-and-after-school program, a religious education program involving 1,400 students, and an active physical education program, all providing avenues for GMU nursing students to meet the goals and course objectives. The goals for this clinical are health promotion, disease prevention through education, therapeutic communications, and health assessments of individuals, families, and small groups.

The next phase in creating the GMU/Nativity Partnership for HEALTH was a meeting with the pastor, one of the pastoral ministers, the school principal, and school nurse. At this meeting potential activities were outlined, and specific implementation strategies were designed. Two major priorities were identified, the first being the need to market the partnership and the second to assess the health promotion and needs of the faith community. These priorities were accomplished simultaneously. The faculty member, who was also a member of this faith community, and I described the partnership to the congregation during each Mass two weekends before the clinical rotation was to begin. A needs assessment survey

Table 12-1 Needs Assessment Survey

Church of the Nativity of Our Lord/GMU Partnership for Health

Sponsored by:
George Mason University College of Nursing and Health Science
Joanne Langan, RN, MSN, Coordinator of Clinical Placement
Margaret "Peggy" Moss, RN, MSN, Instructor

Clinical Nursing is a component of the undergraduate nursing program at George Mason University. Ten third-year nursing students will be participating in a parish health clinic at the Church of the Nativity of Our Lord, Burke, Va. The students will be under the supervision of an instructor who is a licensed professional nurse and has a master's degree in nursing. A variety of health services for people of all ages will be provided by the students and their instructor. Specific programs and services offered will be based on the following survey. We would appreciate you completing this survey and returning it to the bright green and gold box located at the Church vestibule *no later than January 26, 2002. Thank you.*

DEMOGRAPHIC INFORMATION

1. Your age range:
___ 8–12 years
___ 13–19 years
___ 20–40 years
___ 41–64 years
___ over 65 years

Gender:
___ Male
___ Female

2. What is your cultural/ethnic orientation?
_____

3. Marital status?
___ Single
___ Married
___ Divorced
___ Widowed

Please mark (X) the program topics that would interest you.

4. In what ways do you think a parish health program might be helpful in your congregation?
___ Personal health counseling
___ Health education
___ Blood pressure screening
___ Visiting the sick
___ Training health volunteers
___ Health referrals
___ Support groups
___ Other (please specify)

5. Family life and relationships
___ Dealing with parents
___ Peers — when to say "no"
___ Multigenerational relationships
___ Blended families
___ Single parenting
___ Parenting issues: (infants/young children/teens/adult children) Please specify:
_____

Continued

Table 12–1 *Continued*   **Needs Assessment Survey**

6. Healthy living
- ____ Healthy eating
- ____ Smoking/substance abuse
- ____ Activity/exercise
- ____ Relaxation techniques
- ____ Time management
- ____ Stress management
- ____ Safety at school and play
- ____ Infant safety
- ____ Safety for elderly people
- ____ Cholesterol education

7. Understanding
- ____ Feelings: happy/angry/hostile/disappointed
- ____ Sexuality
- ____ Steroid use
- ____ Midlife changes
- ____ Preparing for retirement
- ____ Living the retired life
- ____ Change and loss
- ____ Dealing with loss
- ____ Caregiving and aging (parents/relatives)
- ____ Newborn care
- ____ Hospice
- ____ Living wills/advanced directives

8. Health related
- ____ Cardiopulmonary resuscitation (CPR)
- ____ First aid
- ____ Cancer prevention and detection
- ____ Hypertension
- ____ Diabetes
- ____ Acquired immunodeficiency syndrome/human immunodeficiency syndrome (AIDS/HIV)
- ____ Alzheimer's disease
- ____ Prenatal care
- ____ Women's health
- ____ Postpartum follow-up visits
- ____ Osteoporosis
- ____ Arthritis
- ____ Pain management
- ____ Eating disorders

What other topics interest you? _____

_____

_____

If you are interested in a home visit or individual health counseling, please give your name and telephone number.

Name: _____ Telephone: H _____ W _____

Thank You

(Table 12–1) was inserted into the bulletin, and some were collected after each of these same Masses. There was also a bright green decorated box with the GMU logo on it placed in the vestibule for further collection. I was available after each Mass to meet with parishioners and answer questions.

Eleven-hundred surveys were distributed, and a total of 141 were completed and returned. Parishioners were asked to check health-care topics of interest and to indicate their preferences for health-related programs and activities. A frequency count (Table 12–2) provided the data for possible activities and educational programs.

The results of the needs assessment survey became the framework for the activities, educational programs, and special projects throughout the semester. Three families requested our services for home visits, and we were able to accommodate each of them.

One major lesson learned was that the inclusion of sexuality, under the heading of understanding, resulted in five letters of disapproval and questions regarding subject material, instructor qualifications, and intended audience. These parents indicated that they should be the sole teachers of sexuality. The school nurse, who happens to be a registered nurse and member of this faith community, was asked to correspond in writing to these five parents. Three other respondents crossed out sexuality, which we interpreted as an exclusion decision. Because of the sensitivity regarding sexuality, I would choose not to include that topic in a needs assessment survey for a faith community. Another lesson learned was to place the survey, with a pencil, in the pew and encourage parishioners to complete them at the end of the Mass. They could then turn in the survey as well as ask any questions or seek additional information. I believe this facilitated a better survey return rate. I would also recommend including nursing students in the data collection if possible.

Partnership in Action

It was time to begin this new adventure. Students were anxious, inquisitive, excited, ready, and willing to enter this fertile environment. Our first orientation session was held at GMU, where all the concerns and logistics regarding this new clinical site were addressed. This was an excellent time for the instructor to allay fears and any misconceptions regarding nursing in a faith community. A student inquired, "Are any special characteristics required for this particular clinical site?" The answer is, students need to posses those characteristics required for community-based nursing in any setting, including autonomy, flexibility, effective communications skills, self-confidence, and a strong knowledge base. Students do not have to be from the religion of the faith community where they are assigned; however, they do need to possess a degree of spiritual maturity to function effectively (Abbott 1998). Students do need to be mindful that our clients are all very spiritual. If the students are comfortable with praying, they may do so with the clients. Many of the clients will end their visit with the students by saying, "Thank you and God bless you." I have found that students enjoy this ending and will reply in the same manner. The agenda for this orientation includes introductions to clinical group and instructor, review of the syllabus and required assignments, directions to the site and clinical hours, managing lunch, and safety of valuables. In addition, we discuss appropriate dress, nametag, and lab coat with GMU patch for home visits. Logistics like phone trees, parking, and how to manage lunch and safety of valuables are addressed as well. Students are

Table 12-2

Frequency Count for Activities and Programs

Topics Selected	Frequency
Activity/Exercise	71
Hypertension/Heart Disease	69
Woman's Health	61
Safety for the Elderly	55
CPR	49
Cholesterol Education	45
Healthy Living	44

asked to suggest activities, and results of the needs assessment survey are shared. Time is allotted for questions and answers.

A daily clinical log is required, which will facilitate applications of theory and nursing diagnosis to clinical practice. Students are encouraged to express their thoughts, feelings, experiences, concerns, and special moments along this journey in community-based nursing. Their first log entry should address the questions in Box 12–1.

The first day of clinical arrived, and I found myself excited and happy to be able to share this new clinical site with the students. Nativity provided a welcome coffee, and the significant members of our partnership (principal, pastoral ministers, school nurse, and before-and-after-school coordinator) as well as the secretaries and receptionist were there to meet and greet the students. Each one presented a short description of his or her particular role within this faith community and offered suggestions as to ways the students could be involved. The pastor was unable to be present at the coffee, but he came later in the day to meet and welcome the students. The students felt welcome and relaxed. One of them remarked, "Everyone seems really glad to have us here, and there are so many opportunities for us to meet our objectives." Next, a tour of the facility was provided and additional introductions completed.

The rest of the morning was spent discussing possible activities, selecting home-visit partners for the semester, reviewing available home-visit clients, sharing ideas for teaching projects, assessing age-group preferences, and reviewing specific requests from the needs assessment surveys. One of the unique aspects of nursing in a faith community is the fact that nothing is either included or excluded; rather the activities are derived from human need (Joel 1999). Students are encouraged to develop their projects and educational programs and to select clients based on their own personal strengths and interests.

According to the needs assessment survey, blood pressure screening was important to the congregation. The first activity agreed upon was to implement a weekly blood pressure screening clinic, after a regularly scheduled daily Mass, for 2 hours in the church vestibule with two nursing students participating. The need to announce this event was paramount. A request was submitted for permission to add this to the announcements for the upcoming weekend services. Permission was granted. A poster was constructed and placed in the church vestibule, and an announcement was written for the weekly bulletin. All of the students were eager to participate and agreed to begin the following week. What else might we need for this event? It was decided that a handout should be made on which we would record the parishioner's blood pressure and give to them. One student volunteered to construct a poster with facts about blood pressure. Another student volunteered to make a banner on her computer to be placed on top of the table. Everyone agreed that the following clinical day we would have a mini-clinic and practice blood pressure readings on each other. Students would bring their stethoscopes and sphygmomanometers. I distributed a calendar for the 4 months we would be at Nativity, and students immediately began to sign up for these important activities and record deadlines.

Box 12-1 Learning Exercise for Faculty Use

Log Entry Guide

Please answer the following questions in your log prior to the first day of clinical.

What are some of your assumptions about nursing in a faith community?

What are your expectations of this clinical experience?

What are your expectations of the clinical faculty?

State one personal objective for this experience.

A second activity to be considered was to have space in the weekly church bulletin to present a short column addressing a health fact. The students brainstormed possible subjects, topics, ideas, format, title, and other logistics for producing this column. Students realized this was an excellent method to disseminate information and supplement knowledge requested in the needs assessment survey. A unanimous decision was made among the students to participate in this activity. The column would be called Nativity/GMU Partnership for HEALTH. Each student signed up for a specific date and topic. Each column was checked before it was submitted. The columns would either be delivered a week in advance or faxed to the editor by a specific deadline. The students agreed to begin this activity the following week. Another date added to the calendar of events!

Another activity discussed was the before-and-after-school program. The before-school program starts at 7, and the after-school program hours are 3 to 6. This is a very appealing alternative for make-up hours if a student misses a clinical day for one reason or another. The coordinator, who is a registered nurse, is very supportive of nursing students utilizing this population for teaching projects and activities. Students who wanted to participate registered, and others were aware of this as a viable option.

The clinical conference revolved around a discussion regarding terms we would be using in this particular clinical site that might not be used in other sites:

- spirituality
- "new age" holistic care
- parish nurse
- congregations
- church
- mosque
- temple
- synagogue
- pastoral care
- ministers of health
- Shalom

The students complete the assignment (Box 12–2):

> **Box 12-2** Learning Exercise for Faculty Use
>
> ## Clinical Conference Activity
>
> On a separate sheet of paper define the term spirituality and what it means to you. Then choose three other terms from the list above to define. Twenty minutes will be allowed for this exercise. First the students shared their perceptions of spirituality, and then we discussed the other terms. This activity usually elicits many different responses and is an excellent way to begin to get to know the students.

The final activity was a windshield survey. The students were encouraged to go in pairs to investigate the neighborhood surrounding Nativity. I refer to this as a "getting to know the community" activity. They were to locate and record the addresses for the nearest fire and police stations, health-care facility, hospital, and library. They were to locate the nearest shopping center and make a note regarding the nature of the stores within that area. They should also know the location of the nearest gas station and pharmacy. This exercise assisted them in becoming familiar with their surroundings, an essential for all student nurses in a community setting. They shared this information the next clinical day.

Planning, planning, and more planning is the nature of the initial days at this new clinical site. The second day began with discussion of the windshield survey and the realization that a major health-care facility was at least 15 miles away. Students were surprised at this fact and many admitted that they had never really thought about this issue.

A mini blood pressure screening clinic was organized. All students were able to practice on each other; teachers and the school and church office staff volunteered to participate as well. The students exhibited the banner, poster, and blood pressure record that they had developed for our approval. The students enjoyed experiencing a real-life test of their knowledge. The responsibility of preparing and disseminating health information drew on their professional values of integrity, accuracy, and honesty. They witnessed the demands of assessing and documenting health data correctly and protecting the confidentiality of client information

Chapter 12 | Teaching Students in a Faith Community

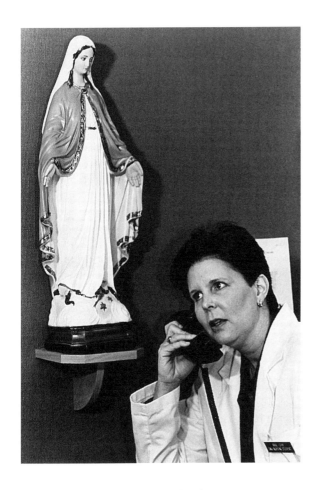

and learning, teaching strategies, and learning in the three domains. I also discuss the assessment of learning needs including learner characteristics that affect learning.

The science teacher, who is a nurse, approached me regarding nursing students teaching anatomy and physiology to sixth graders. The class is usually 45 minutes in length, and there are 29 children. I presented this proposal to my students, and they all welcomed the opportunity to participate. The students agreed this would not be the major teaching project but a mini teaching project. The 10 systems of the body were listed, and each student selected one, a date to present, and an observation date. Observational experiences accompanied by guidelines can be an extremely beneficial teaching strategy. The purpose of an observational session is to observe classroom environment, classroom equipment (overhead, a projection screen, charts), strategies of teaching being implemented, conduct of the teacher, discipline used (if any), and attention span of the students. Students were to have their teaching plan completed and approved 1 week in advance. Each student also submitted four test questions to be used by the science teacher. I accompanied and evaluated each student as they taught the science class; this was an invaluable experience and teaching opportunity. Working to plan and deliver the classes provided experiential learning that served the students well. They learned a great deal about themselves. It also resulted in a great deal of creativity and teaching talent being generated on the part of the GMU nursing students.

This particular clinical site has a full-time school nurse. She offered to have each student spend an observational session with her. All of the students welcomed the opportunity to examine the role and functions of a school nurse. She shared with them all of the state and county guidelines and some of the interesting cases she had cared for in her role as a school nurse. This was the opening year for Nativity School, so everything was brand new and focused on a learning mode. Documentation of care was vital in this setting and provided a student experience that was valuable. My students were amazed at how well the nurse knew all 250 children and their current health status. She was also available as a consultant and resource for teaching projects.

The two pastoral ministers shared the responsibilities for visiting the ill, the homebound, and the shut-ins and

(Green & Adderley-Kelly 1999). This group was prepared and ready for action.

Teaching is a critical component of one's nursing practice. It is also not a new role for nurses. "In the 1880s Florence Nightingale wrote about sanitation, housing, care of the sick in hospitals, and health teaching. Nightingale recognized that it was not enough for people to be interested in health information, but that the test was whether they practiced it later in their homes" (Whitman et al. 1992, p 6). Every nursing student is required to complete teaching projects. This particular community-based clinical setting had grade school children, teenagers, teachers and staff, parishioners, home-clients, and our student group available for teaching and learning opportunities. During the second week of clinical, I provide a postclinical conference, which reviews the theories of teaching for counseling caretakers, those experiencing serious or terminal illness, and a cadre of lay ministers who distributed communion weekly to parishioners in a variety of settings. They were very willing to share their clients with us. Together we constructed a list of possible clients for the students to visit on a weekly basis for the entire semester. Two students made each home visit; one student had the role of primary student nurse, while the other assumed a secondary role.

The secondary role was that of providing support and pleasant conversation, and being additional eyes and ears. The primary student had the responsibility for ensuring a safe environment, performing basic assessments, and reviewing medications, nutrition, and exercise. She may also have identified additional resources that would benefit the client, while utilizing therapeutic communications. Over the semester, she gathered information to enable her to complete a family assessment. Each weekly home visit lasted about an hour, and many of the clients were seen for 12 to 14 visits, a substantial amount of time to positively impact a client's health. The first two visits were spent establishing rapport, beginning to gather information about the client, performing a safety check of the environment, and discussing what the expectations would be for subsequent visits. Each student was responsible for keeping a detailed log of each visit. If for any reason a client needed to be referred to another agency or physician, there was a referral sheet available (Table 12–3).

Home visits were anxiety producing! Students had many questions and concerns regarding this assignment. Some of the questions were, "What will I say? How will I act? Will my client like me? Will my client ask me questions I don't know? How do I begin to examine my client? What equipment will I need?" These fears and concerns were addressed through group discussion, role-playing exercises, and a video. I assured the students that I would accompany each of them on their first home visit. I shared my previous visit with their client, and the pastoral ministers came and shared the knowledge they possessed regarding the clients. The students viewed a video of a simulated home visit in their first clinical laboratory at GMU. I showed a video," The Parish Nurse: A Ministry to Older Adults," which was obtained from the International Parish Nurse Resource Center located in Park Ridge, Illinois. This video presented parish nurses working in urban, rural, and suburban settings with a focus on the needs of the older adult in these settings. Through hearing from the older adults themselves, an understanding of the roles of personal health counselor, health educator, developer of support groups, trainer of volunteers, and liaison with the community, the concept of parish nursing came alive. A lengthy discussion followed the video and students reported they had a much better idea regarding the role and functions of the parish nurse. Decisions were made and a client-student roster was produced. Another event was placed on the calendar.

Students were concerned about completing physical assessments, for they hadn't done a great many of them since the fall semester. Their concerns led me to obtain a Springhouse Video, "Assessing the Adult: Head to Toe," which shows how to perform a complete physical assessment efficiently and confidently. The video is 55 minutes long, and students were encouraged to take it home and use it as a review. Over the next few weeks eight of the students checked it out.

One of the students had asked about equipment required for a home visit. We decided as a group that equipment was needed, and it would be best to organize and assemble a nursing bag. Next we brainstormed what should be included in this nursing bag. The students decided that it should contain pens, pencil, paper, stethoscope, sphygmomanometer, scissors, flashlight, a few pairs of disposable gloves, a Northern Virginia map, drug book, and a pocket assessment book (if they owned one). In addition, students carried three file cards, one with the client's address, phone number, and directions to their home, another with the instructor's beeper and car phone number, and a third with Nativity's main phone number.

The following letter is one family member's description of nursing students' home visits:

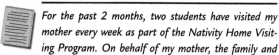

For the past 2 months, two students have visited my mother every week as part of the Nativity Home Visiting Program. On behalf of my mother, the family and myself, I want to thank and highly commend both students for their attitudes of openness, readiness to help and serve, and for the joy they brought their "patient." Although my mother is very hard of hearing and her main language is Spanish, this was not an impediment for Diane and Angela to patiently communicate with her

Table 12–3

Referral Form

Church of the Nativity of Our Lord/GMU Partnership for Health

To:
From:
Date:

Church of the Nativity of Our Lord/GMU Partnership for Health is a collaborative project between the Church of the Nativity of Our Lord and George Mason University College of Nursing and Health Science. The project focuses on health promotion and disease prevention. The students and their nursing instructor are responsible for activities, including health teaching, health screening, and home visiting.

The following parishioner has been assessed by a student and is being referred to you for evaluation.

Parishioner: _____

Problem: _____
_____
_____
_____
_____

Student: _____

Instructor: _____

If you have any questions, please call Margaret "Peggy" Moss at (123) 456-7890.

---

and share with her an extremely enjoyable visit. The student nurses instructed her on her medications, diet, and nutrition; took her blood pressure; massaged her legs; helped her care for a bed sore that appeared; and listened to all my mother's stories of her life. All this was done in every visit with the best disposition. We are very grateful. Please accept our highest praise for these two lovely junior nursing students.

Safety is an important objective in all clinical settings and rotations. Safety extends to all members of the health-care team, students and clients. Student safety is critical in home visiting. In most cases I am able to make a home visit prior to the semester beginning; if I don't then I must rely on input from the pastoral minister who has recently seen the client. I attended the first home visit with each student to teach by example and be a role model. As mentioned earlier, students made home visits in pairs. The students always called before going out on a visit; this serves to let the client know they are on their way, and allows the client to relay any additional information or needs.

It is imperative that students know who will be in the home other than the client. Some of our clients were unable to move about well and students needed to let themselves in by accessing a key or the door being left unlocked. Students would then lock the door before leaving. I always have a set of file cards with the client's name, address, and phone number as well as directions to their home, in my car and in my nursing bag. I rely on my beeper and car phone to keep me accessible and in communication with my students. There are days when six of the students will be out and about at the same time, and it is important that assistance, if needed, is only a phone call or beeper away.

A health fair for the elementary school children was also a great idea! Health fairs are an excellent venue for impacting large numbers of participants on a variety of health-promotion, disease-prevention topics and activities. It is a huge undertaking and requires hours of planning. Ours took the whole semester to organize. Initially the students made the decision to consider this teaching option. It was quickly realized that to have a successful health fair, all students would have to participate, and cooperation and collaboration would be essential ingredients. Students would develop a booth of their own for the fair. Students could recruit professionals from the health arena to assist them and actually work the booth, or just contribute advice and resources. During the first discussion we reviewed possible booth topics, explored resources, examined the calendar of events for school activities, and analyzed some of the logistics of such an undertaking. It was decided that the theme of the fair would be children's health. A part of each clinical day was spent organizing the fair.

Suggestions for planning and implementing the health fair included obtaining a letter from Nativity's school principal supporting the nursing students' efforts to obtain free samples of products to distribute to the school children, for example yogurt, pretzels, or tooth paste. Requesting these free samples needs to be done early for it can take a few weeks for them to arrive. Always have the samples sent to the facility. Get the event on the school

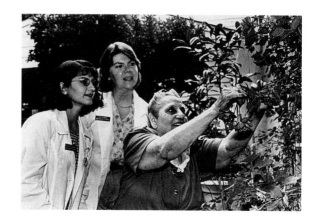

calendar early. Think about making posters to place around the school. Check on actual space for the fair, make a mock set-up of the room, and measure the spaces. Request the tables and chairs needed, and determine the expectations of the environmental staff for the day of event. Need to open the school earlier? Need assistance with take down? Need extra electricity? Can you close off the event room for lunch or breaks? What will you do for lunch? All of these questions need to be answered in the planning sessions. Students should be given time to go to the library or the craft store to purchase necessary supplies. Will you need handouts duplicated? Who will do this? Who will pay for them? Maybe the school will let you use its copier if you supply the paper? How will the cost of doing this fair be decided and divided? What is a reasonable cost? Best to try to do it as cost-effectively as possible by requesting donations. Will you have food snacks for the children? You will need to get a list of students with food allergies and those on special diets if food is to be offered. Planning, planning, and more planning will make this event a success for everyone. I usually supply snacks for the nursing students that they can enjoy between classes, for it is a very long, tiring day. But the health fair is one of the highlights of this clinical experience.

The second "getting to know the community" activity was to visit a community health-resource organization for the purpose of learning the mission, goals, and objectives of this organization. The students also obtained free samples of available teaching aids and resources (literature, posters, displays, video checklist, and equipment) as well as lists of possible speakers and references.

Organizations we used included American Heart Association, American Cancer Society, Dental Association, Lung Association, Alzheimer Association, County Center for Aging, National Osteoporosis Association, National Dairy Council, County Center for Children, National Hospice Foundation, and American Diabetes Association. All of these are within a 20-mile radius of this clinical setting. Students shared their experiences and resources the following clinical day. This was the beginning of developing a resource file or box (Box 12–3 and 12–4).

All schools have physical education (PE) programs, and this presents another area of possible involvement for students. When I arrived at Nativity, the principal mentioned that the PE program needed some assistance, for the teacher was a new graduate and was having difficulty implementing the Presidential Physical Fitness Program. By the time the clinical had started, the PE teacher had terminated. The principal inquired if the nursing students could plan, implement, and test the Presidential Physical Fitness Program. I explained that it would be up to the nursing students to decide, and that the program would require some investigation and discussion. After careful consideration, four students agreed to administer, teach, and test this program for grades two through eight. National headquarters was immediately notified, and records, requirements, and brochures were sent. The classes were divided into upper and lower divisions, folders with class rosters organized, a meeting with the PE substitute teacher arranged, class schedules rearranged to accommodate nursing students' availability, and all students began to practice the V-sits and chin pulls. Nursing students were allowed to wear sweat suits for teaching, and I gave them all a whistle for control. This activity was a marvelous experience for all who participated. Nursing students learned a great deal about the normal growth and development of children of all ages and the importance of limit setting and consistency in dealing with them. The program was completed and awards were ordered; a small number of the students actually earned the highest honor but everyone was given a certificate and patch for participation. The nursing students planned an award ceremony, and each student was called forward to receive his or her award. I am sure that next year many of the students will work even harder, for the principal allowed the nursing students to order special T-shirts for all those who

---

Box 12-3   Learning Exercise for Faculty Use

Brainstorming Community Resources

If a stranger moving into your community were to inquire about its health-care agencies, which would you list?

Would students list local churches?

Would you have listed local churches before reading this chapter?

If local churches were not listed, ask...

What about the church? Is it really a health agency?

Can you list at least four church activities or programs that might be seen as contributing to health and wellness of a congregation?

Box 12-4   Learning Exercise for Faculty Use

Identification of Community Resources

Have each student list at least five health-resource organizations in your community.

Then make a master list including addresses and phone number of the organizations.

Each student should visit one of these organizations.

made presidential honors. Four students were adequate to complete the program but six would have been even better, for the extra student in each division could have been a recorder and in charge of the paper work.

One issue worth mentioning is the weather. We start this clinical in late January and during the next 2 months the weather could complicate PE classes and accomplishing our goals. There always needs to be a plan B and a place to implement it. This is not always convenient for most facilities; therefore the schedule of events must be carefully planned. Despite these limitations, I would highly recommend that if utilizing a school site, getting involved with the PE program is worthwhile.

The clinical was now well under way. Students' calendars were full of activities and deadlines for the semester. Ideas for teaching projects were being suggested, assessed, planned, and formalized. Students would take advantage of the various populations at this clinical site for implementation of teaching projects. One student decided to offer a presentation for the teachers and staff. She produced a written survey to determine the topic of interest (Table 12–4). They chose a stress-management program.

Table 12-4

Teacher Survey

Church of the Nativity of Our Lord/GMU Partnership for Health

Below are some health-related topics being considered for development into educational programs specifically aimed towards teachers. We would like your input as to which topics you would like us to present as a part of the Church of the Nativity of Our Lord/GMU Partnership for HEALTH promotion program. Comments, additions, suggestions, etc. are more than welcome.

Please select from the following, the topics you are most interested in. You may select more than one topic.

____ First Aid

____ Recognizing the signs of abuse

____ Positive self-esteem building in children

____ Stress management

____ Classroom safety

____ Healthy snacks for healthy children

Comments/Additions/Suggestions _____

_____

_____

_____

_____

Thank you!

The student did an excellent job of providing a 45-minute stress-reduction workshop. From the quiet music, mildly-scented burning candles, hot-spiced tea, homemade sweet bread, low lighting and comfortable chairs, the student was able to introduce various techniques for relaxation. Stress-reduction exercises and techniques were practiced. She engaged the participants through a sharing session on techniques they utilize to reduce stress. She also gave them handouts with additional suggestions for reducing and managing stress. There were 15 participants, and they all appeared much more relaxed at the end of the workshop. It was agreed that teaching could be a very stressful job. One teacher commented on her way out, "I feel so relaxed now; I think I will just go home."

"Germ Busters," " Stranger Danger," " 911," " What is Depression?," "Hugs not Drugs," "Personal Hygiene," "Parts is Parts," and "Importance of Hand Washing" are just a few titles of teaching projects presented. One student wanted to teach a basic hygiene and normal growth and development class to fifth graders. To do this, a permission slip was sent to the parents, and only the students with a positive response attended (Table 12–5). Only one parent refused. These teaching projects were all constructed for various classes at Nativity School. Most could be taught in 20 to 30 minutes. Students selected topics, wrote objectives for the teaching-learning activity, and then approached the classroom teacher for permission to execute their plan, as well as to observe the class. Students did one-on-one client teaching regarding medications, diabetes, foot care, nutrition, exercise requirements, and alcohol awareness, to mention a few. Active learning strategies are incorporated into all teaching-learning projects as well as use of community resources and handouts to enhance and reinforce learning.

TEACHING STRATEGIES

Extensive faculty-student conferences provided the avenue for sharing experiences and problem-solving strategies each day. Members of the partnership were consulted as appropriate when problems surfaced, and they often participated in the decision-making process. As the students and faculty consulted with each other, shared ideas, and evaluated and planned strategies, critical thinking was promoted.

Clinical conference is a major strategy used to promote student learning. At this faith community site students were involved in many activities, which took place in different settings. It was very important that we came together for sharing of individual experiences and monitoring of progress on group projects. It was also a time for didactic teaching such as a conference on teaching and learning theories and principles, and learning styles, as well as barriers to teaching and learning. Box 12–5 illustrates a case study that could be used in conference.

Experiential learning is learning not likely to be forgotten. Providing opportunities for collaboration with other professionals is an essential component of students' work in this setting. The students' experience with the school nurse was extremely informative. They viewed a career option, and because this particular nurse had worked in occupational health nursing for 20 years, she readily shared her experiences. She was an excellent resource. Coordination of activities with the pastor and pastoral ministers was valuable to the students' learning too.

Another teaching strategy, the clinical log, requires a daily entry. It is an invaluable learning activity. The log provides an opportunity for students to document their responses to clinical experiences. The log will facilitate applications of theory and nursing diagnosis to clinical practice. The purpose of the log is to provide an avenue for expressing feelings and engaging in a dialogue with

Table 12-5

Parental Permission Slip

Dear Parent,

The GMU Nursing Students will be teaching a class on Basic Hygiene and Normal Growth and Development to 5th grade on Wednesday, May 5.

To participate each student must have a signed permission slip.

I do/do not give _____ permission to participate in Basic Hygiene Class.

(Child's Name) _____

_____
Parent's Signature   Date

> **Box 12-5** Learning Exercise for Faculty Use
>
> ### Case Study
>
> During the 4th week of the clinical at Nativity two nursing students were visiting Mrs. B, a 78-year-old that lives in a small apartment complex for senior citizens. Mrs. B suffers from hypertension and depression, and she had a triple coronary artery bypass 6 months ago. She lives alone in a very nicely decorated one-bedroom apartment. She does have a daughter who lives nearby. On this particular visit, the students were reviewing the medications ordered for Mrs. B. The client was familiar with many of the medications but others she wasn't knowledgeable about at all. The medications included digitoxin, lasix, baby aspirin, lovastatin, capton, K-Dur and xoloft. During the visit Mrs. B confided in the students that most days she only took half of each medication for she feared her new health insurance wouldn't pay for her prescriptions. Mrs. B said, "I'm not sure I need all this medication anyway. What do you think?"
>
> 1. How would you answer this question?
>
> 2. What resources would you employ to assist Mrs. B?
>
> 3. What further teaching needs to be implemented?
>
> 4. Would you expect this situation to be common among the geriatric population?

teachers about them (Oermann & Gaberson 1998). It assists in monitoring the student's progress and is extremely helpful with clinical evaluation.

Evaluation

Formative and summative evaluations were conducted via conferences, instructor supervision and participation during home visits, feedback from members of the partnership and parishioners, review of journals, and formal evaluation of teaching projects. Activities were modified based on formative evaluations. Each student evaluated himself or herself on all teaching projects and activities. Together we arrived at the clinical grade.

Suggestions

Faith community nurses have the potential to reduce the cost of health care and improve the quality of life in the next century by focusing on the prevention of disease before the need for expensive treatment. Faith community nurses are documenting their outcomes and, with them, instances of cases in which faith community nurses' interventions have potentially resulted in substantial cost savings to the federal government through averted Medicare expenses. Theoretically, Rydholm (1997) estimated a cost saving of $400,000 to Medicare through 600 home visits made by parish nurses. Half of these estimates were related to scenarios where caregivers were sustained to facilitate ongoing home care and the other half were related to signs and symptoms warranting prompt attention. Advocacy, referral, assistance finding, active listening, and supportive education efforts served to overcome major stumbling blocks to access for those elders and their caregivers who felt physically and emotionally isolated or overwhelmed by their situation (Rydholm 1997).

Faith community nursing efforts to articulate outcomes needs to be expanded. Nursing students need to be grounded in outcome language if they are to be empowered to articulate their scope of practice in this crucial age that threatens to devalue holistic practice. The only way to capture the extent of the impact on client health is to incorporate outcome data into a documentation system. The system needs to be easy and clear. The International Parish Nurse Resource Center (IPNRC) in collaboration with Advocate Parish Nursing Services is one of seven test sites to test and enhance the Nursing Outcomes Classification System (NOC). NOC is a classification system of nursing-sensitive patient outcomes, which includes the spiritual dimension of care. The results of this testing will provide evidence to support outcomes with a more whole person perspective.

There is very little published research in parish nursing. This is attributed to lack of funding, newness of

Table 12-6

Resources

ORGANIZATIONS

The International Nurse Resource Center

205 W. Touky, Suite 124

Park Ridge, Ill. 60068

(800) 556-5368

Health Ministries Association

P.O. Box 7853

Huntington Beach, Ca. 92646

Phone (714) 965-0085

BOOKS

Solari-Twadell PA et al. (Eds.) (1990). Parish nursing: The developing practice. Park Ridge, IL: National Parish Nurse Resource Center.

Solari-Twadell PA & McDermott MA (1999). Parish nursing. Thousand Oaks, CA: Sage Publishers.

Solari-Twadell PA, et al. (Eds.) (1994). Assuring Viability for the future: Guideline development for parish nurse education programs. Park Ridge, OIL: National Parish Nurse Resource Center.

VIDEOS

The Healing Team, An Introduction to Health Ministry and Parish Nursing. Produced by Bay Area Health Ministries, (415) 221-3693, www.bahm.org.

The Parish Nurse: A ministry to older adults. Available from the International Parish Nurse Resource Center.

Parish Nurses: Reclaiming their joy. Available from the International Parish Nurse Resource Center.

Yours Are the Hands, Parish Nurse Program, Resurrection Health Care, (773) 774-8650.

ARTICLES

Abbott B (1998). Parish nursing. Home Healthcare Nurse, 16 (4), 265–267.

Penner S & Galloway-Lee B (1997). Parish nursing: Opportunities in community health. Home Care Provider 2 (5), 244–249.

Rydholm L (1997). Patient-focused care in parish nursing. Holistic Nursing Practice 11 (3), 47–60.

Schank MJ, et al. (1996). Parish nursing: Ministry of healing. Geriatric Nursing 17(1), 11–13.

Weis D et al. (1997). Health care delivery in faith communities: The parish nurse model. Public Health Nursing 14(6), 368–372.

specialty, and a lack of shared understanding of the concept (Martin 1996). This is fertile ground open to all of us who participate in nursing in a faith community.

Nursing in a faith community is emerging as a viable response to the multiple and complex problems that constitute the crisis that this nation is experiencing in health care.

It is proving to be an excellent clinical site for nursing students whose focus is on health promotion, disease prevention, development of self-care capacity and holistic care. GMU students had an immense impact on the health status of this faith community. To quote a student, "Faith communities have it all!" I must agree, and I feel extremely privileged to have had the opportunity to develop this community-based site.

References

Abbott, B (1998). Parish nursing. Homecare Healthc Nurse 16(4), 265-267.

Baron, R (Ed.) (1993). Jefferson the man: In his own words. Washington, DC: Library of Congress.

Bergquist, D & King, J (1994). Parish nursing: A conceptual framework. J Holist Nurs 12(2), 155-170.

Biddix, V & Brown, H (1999). Establishing a parish nurse program. Nurs Health Care Perspect 20(2), 72-75.

Clark, P & Cody, W (1994). Nursing theory-based practice in the home and community: The crux of professional nursing education. Advance Nurs Sci 17(2), 41-53.

Green, P & Adderley-Kelly, B (1999). Partnership for health promotion in an urban community. Nurs Health Care Perspect 20(2), 76-81.

Joel, L (1999). Parish nursing: As old as faith communities. AJN (8), 7.

Martin, L (1996). Parish nursing: Keeping body and soul together. Canadian Nurse 92(1), 25-28.

Oermann, MH & Gaberson, KB (1998). Evaluation and testing in nursing education. New York: Springer.

Rydholm, L (1997). Patient-focused care in parish nursing. Holist Nurs Pract 11(3), 47-60.

Solari-Twadell, PA et al. (Eds.) (1990). Parish nursing: The developing practice. Park Ridge, Ill: National Parish Nurse Resource Center.

Solari-Twadell, PA & McDermott, MA (Eds.) (1999). Parish nursing: Promoting whole person health within faith communities. Thousand Oaks, Calif: Sage.

Weis, D et al. (1997). Health care delivery in faith communities: The parish nurse model. Public Health Nurs 14(6), 368-372.

Whitman, N et al. (1992). Teaching in Nursing Practice. Norwalk, Conn: Appleton-Century-Crofts.

INDEX

A
AACN. *See* American Association of Colleges of Nursing
Activities
   frequency count of, 166
   list of, 9
Acute-care settings, 77
   assignments in, 79
   emphasis in, 79
   goal in, 79
Adult day care, 95
Adult health, 22
Advocate Parish Nursing Services, 176
Affiliation agreements, 4, 10-11
Agencies
   contacting, 7-8
   regulations of, 65-66, 76
   rules of, 65-66
Agency-university partnership, 4
Altruism, 20
Ambiguities, 71
American Association of Colleges of Nursing (AACN), 18, 41
Applicants, paperwork required, 19
Assessments, 5-6
   of family, 104
   ongoing, 78
   of students, 77
Assisted living, 95
ASTHMA PROJECT, 111
Autonomy, 60

B
Bag techniques, 64
BAP. *See* Bits and Pieces
Behavior, non-judgmental, 20
Beveled Edges, 37-38
Bits and Pieces (BAP), 55-57
Black Peer Counseling Program, 129
Bolton Model, 150

C
Calendar, 80-81
Campus clinical, 121-122
   challenges of, 136
   confidentiality agreement, 123
   evaluation, 135-136
   family assessment, 134-135
   follow-up, 135-136
   ground work, 122-123
   health promotion survey, 129
   implementation, 123-136
   one-time projects, 124
   operations base, 122
   orientation to, 123-124
   pitfalls, 133-135
   problems, 133-135
   rotation grid, 127
   semester commitments, 134
   student projects for, 124-125
   student supervision in, 126-133
   time log, 128
   time usage, 125-126, 134
   unit evaluation, 135
Case studies, 31-32
Case Western Reserve, 150
CBC. *See* Community-based issues, curriculum
Children, care of underserved, 109
CHN. *See* Community health nursing
Church of Nativity. *See* Nativity
Clinical activities, 77-79
Clinical agencies
   assumptions for, 72
   evaluation forms, 86-88
Clinical debriefing, 46
Clinical evaluation, 82-83

Clinical experiences, 73-77
Clinical family concept, 146
Clinical instructors, 89
Clinical logs, 44
Clinical nursing education, 147
Clinical placement coordinator, 7
Clinical Post-Conference Learning Environment Survey (CPCLES), 47
Clinical rotations, 6
   acute-care, 72-73
   in community-based experiences, 71
Clinical settings, 86-90
Clinical sites, 72
Clinical supervision, 12-14
College campuses, 121. *See also* Campus clinical
Commitment, 21
Communication
   chain, 102
   by faculty, 78-79
   home visits and, 55-57
   lack of, 15
   letter, 58
   skills, 25-26, 117
   strategies, 102-103
   therapeutic, 104
Community
   activities, 102
   agency staff, 76
   assessment of, 64-65
   health fair, 117
   knowledge of, 58
   partnerships, 4-6
Community-based issues
   agency assignments, 79
   care *vs.* hospital stays, 61
   clinical sites, 73
   content leveling, 72
   curriculum, 18, 41
   junior-level course, 73
   nursing, 4
Community-based sites
   choosing, 3-4
   contracting for, 3-4
   development, 110-113
   faculty applications in, 110-115
   securing, 6
Community health nursing (CHN), 4
Community setting
   content of, 25
   knowledge of, 25
   unstructured, 71-72
Compassion, 23-24
Competency, 21-22
Composition research, 32-33
Confidence, 22-23
Confidentiality, 20, 77
   in campus clinical, 123
   statement, 123
Conscience, 24-25
Consultation, 11-14
Continuum of care, 89
Contract person, 16
Contracts, 14-16
   pitfalls in, 15-16
   student/instructor, 83-84
Course evaluation forms, 85
Course Report Form (CRF), 87
Course syllabi, 7
CPCLES. *See* Clinical Post-conference Learning Environment Survey
Creativity, 26-27
CRF. *See* Course Report Form
Critical thinking, 22
   exercise, 105
   outcomes, 44
   skills, 83, 117, 119
Crohn's disease, 116
Cultural competence, 20, 27
Cultural diversity, 62
Cultural heritage, 119

D
Debriefing, postclinical, 78
Decision making, in home visits, 60
Dental hygiene, 115
Dependence, 60
Diabetes education, 119
Dignity, 20
Disease prevention, 120
Documentation, of home visits, 66
Drive-through surgery, 61

E
Eating pattern awareness, 131
Elderly persons, 98

Index

Elementary schools
   as community-based site, 109-110
   general concepts, 109-110
   health education in, 115
   home visits in, 114
   teaching strategies for, 116-120
   underserved children in, 109
Employee orientation, 57
Enthusiasm, 26
Essentials of Baccalaureate Education, 41
Ethical issues, 77
Evaluation
   forms of, 85-86
   opportunities for, 77
Evidence, 48
Excellence, 25-27
Experiential learning, 8-10

F
Faculty
   attributes, 95
   consultation with, 11-14
   development for, 18, 89
   selection, 17-27
   status, 16
   supervision, 102-103
Fairfax County Public Health Department, 112-113
Faith communities, 161-162
   activities of, 167
   blood pressure screening clinic, 167
   clinical conference, 175
   clinical log, 167, 175
   community survey, 168
   developing, 163-175
   evaluation, 176
   health fact column, 168
   health fair, 172
   health-resource organizations in, 172-173
   home visits, 170
   needs assessment survey, 164-165
   orientation session, 166
   physical assessments, 170
   referral form, 171
   resources, 177
   safety, 171
   school program, 168
   suggestions, 176
   support, 170
   teacher survey, 174
   teaching projects, 175
   teaching strategies, 175-178
   terminology, 168
   weather impact, 174
Family assessment, 104
   format for, 116-117
Family Development Model, 146
Family development workshops, 89
Family Health Protective Behaviors Assessment Tool, 104
Family privacy, 63
Filing system, 147
Fairfax County Public Health Department, 115
Frustrations, 158

G
George Mason University (GMU), 3-4
GMU. *See* George Mason University
Goals, student-identified, 75
Group solutions, 82
Guidelines for Clinical Supervision, 12

H
Hand washing, 111, 115
Head Start, 75
Health-care
   change in, 61-62
   delivery of, 120
Health fair, 106
Health promotion, 129
   focus of, 118
   projects, 130
   teaching of, 120
Health science guidelines, 12
Healthy living pilot, 132
HHA. *See* Home-health agency
HIV
   population, 27
   services, 17-18, 141
HIV/AIDS community-based site
   case manager mentor, 146
   clinical activity journal, 145
   clinical conference, 145-146
   collaboration, 143-144
   conference times, 144
   disengagement, 143

HIV/AIDS community-based site—*Continued*
  essential knowledge, 140
  establishment phases, 142-146
  evaluation, 143
  faculty, 145, 147
  learning experiences, 141-142
  modules, 142
  network practice, 139-140
  psychological entry, 142
  student supervision, 144-145
  teaching strategies, 145-146
Holistic health care, 162
Home-care setting, 149
Home-health agency (HHA), 159
Home-health clinical
  case study analysis, 157-158
  communication, 151, 153-154
  conferences, 158-159
  faculty flexibility, 154-155
  faculty roles, 151
  interface with providers, 159
  journals, 157
  laboratory simulations, 155-157
  responsibilities in, 150-155
  staff roles, 151
  student partnerships, 159
  student roles, 151
  teaching strategies, 155-159
Home-health settings, 61
Home visits
  communication and, 55-57
  decision making for, 60
  documentation of, 66
  educational information and materials for, 68-69
  in elementary school sites, 114
  in faith communities, 170
  first, 68
  goals, 56, 64
  guidance for, 60
  keys to, 54
  knowledge base, 68
  laboratory practice for, 63-64
  logistics of, 66-67
  mission, 56
  nursing process in, 65-69
  objectives, 56
  organizing for, 67
  planning, 67, 69
  preparing for, 53-54, 63-65
  preplanning, 54-55, 57
  problems with, 68
  process of, 76
  purpose, 67-69
  role modeling for, 69
  safety and, 66-67
  school setting, 114
  senior centers, 99
  settings, 62-63
  simulated, 64
  stages of, 59-60
Hospital discharges, 61
Humor, 26

I
INOVA Juniper Program, 140
In-services, 9
International Parish Nurse Resource Center (IPNRC), 176
Interview session, 18-20
IPNRC. *See* International Parish Nurse Resource Center

J
Journals
  for campus clinical, 126, 130
  entries in, 117-119, 126, 130
  evaluation criteria, 157
  as evaluation tool, 117
  guidelines for, 43
  objectives of, 43
  process, 42-46
  reflective entries, 44-46
  research on, 43-44
Juniper Program, 139-140
  INOVA, 140
Juvenile Diabetes Association, 116

K
Key issues, 74-75

L
Laws, 22
Learning
  activities, 41-42

Index

environment, 82
experiences in senior centers, 104-107
on job (LOJ), 63
needs, 59
perspective, 59-60
portfolios, 48-51
Legal liability, 11
Letters, to community agencies, 57
LGH. *See* Lutheran General Hospital
Life span development, 22
Logistics, of home visits, 66-67
LOJ. *See* Learning, on job
Long-term care, 6
Long-term client, 152
Lutheran General Hospital (LGH), 162

M
Medicare Coverage of Services, 153
Medication administration, 104
Mentoring, 28, 78
MTV, 44
Music, violence in, 44

N
Narratives, 31-32
  using, 117-120
Nativity, 163
  School, 169
Newsletters, 55
Newspaper health column, 133
Nightingale, Florence, 169
NOC. *See* Nursing Outcomes Classification System
Northern Virginia Dental Association, 115
Nurse education, 18
NursEnergy, 75, 125
Nurse practice acts, 22
Nursing
  curriculum changes, 3
  enthusiasm for, 26
  guidelines for, 12
  process framework, 65
  public health, 4
  school setting practice, 115-116
Nursing Outcomes Classification System (NOC), 176
Nutrition, 115

O
Objectives, 7
Office of HIV Services, 141
Orientation, 14
  of agency staff, 73-75
  for faculty, 73-75
  letter, 111
  for students, 74-75
Ostomy Association, 116

P
Paperwork, required of applicants, 19
Parent permission slip, 175
"Parish Nurse: A Ministry to Older Adults," 170
Parish nursing, 162
Parish Nursing: The Developing Practice, 163
Partnerships
  defined, 4
  interdisciplinary, 5
Pathophysiology principles, 22
Peer evaluation, 82-83
Personal boundaries, 62-63
Physical education programs, 173
Policies, 74
Portfolios, 48-51
  assessment of, 44
  best works, 48, 50
  consequences of, 51
  content of, 49
  criteria of, 51
  defined, 48
  evaluation of, 50
  guidelines, 49
  purposes of, 48-49
Postclinical debriefing, 78
Postconferences, 46-51, 64
  benefits, 47
  reflection questions, 47
  research on, 47-48
Preceptors, 150
  benefits of using, 152
  students and, 152-154
Preclinical work, 73-74
Preconferences, 64
Prioritization, 77
Procedures, 74
Professional behavior issues, 76-77
Program frequency count, 166
Public health nursing, 4

R

Read Around, 36, 38
Ready, Set, Go for Good Health, 113
Reflection, 42-46
   as technique and process, 42
   trust in, 42
Regulations, of agency, 65-66
Relationships, mutually beneficial, 9-10
Research, in composition, 32-33
Risk taking, 26
Role modeling, 26
Role-playing, 116
Rules, of agency, 65-66

S

Safety, 76
   common concerns, 67
   in home visits, 66-67
Scenarios, "what if," 64
School setting
   elementary. *See* Elementary schools
   faith community program, 168, 175-178
   home visits, 114
   Nativity, 163, 169
   skills needed in, 110
Science contingency plan, 13
Self-knowledge, 37
Senior centers, 95-98
   clinical activities, 100
   clinical experience requirements, 98
   cultural differences in, 97-98
   developing as clinical site, 98-107
   educational topics for, 106
   family letter, 101
   home visits, 99
   initial visit to, 98
   letters of introduction, 99-100
   planned events, 96
   sample activities in, 96-97
   schedules, 99
   scope of student practice, 103-104
   services offered, 103-104
   student activities, 99-101
   technologies offered, 103-104
Sensitivity, 21
Services
   learning, 8-10
   list of, 9

Settings, unstructured, 72-73
Shadowing, 76
Split sites
   advantages, 7-8
   benefits, 8
   disadvantages, 7-8
   risks, 8
Stories
   composing effective, 35
   data from, 31
   evaluating, 36-38
   group, 35
   guidelines for, 35
   plot of, 35
   reading of, 36
   role in student learning, 29-30
   showcasing, 37-38
   teaching with, 30-32, 35-38
   writing, 36
Storytelling
   in classroom, 33-34
   in clinical experiences, 34
   strategies for, 30, 33-34
Students
   accounting for time of, 101-102
   activities of, 96
   assignments for, 74
   learning of, 79-86
   needs of, 27
   products developed by, 82
   space for, 74
Student health center, 123
Supervision guidelines, 114-115
Surveys
   campus clinical, 129
   community, 168
   CPCLES, 47
   eating pattern awareness, 131
   in faith communities, 164-165, 168, 174
   health promotion, 129
   healthy living pilot, 132
   needs assessment, 164-165
   teacher, 174

T

Teaching
   activities, 41-42
   enthusiasm for, 26

Index

experience, 19
moments, 77
projects, 10
strategies, 30, 104-107
Timeliness, 76
Time management, 77
Timing expectations, 74
Touring, 75
Transportation, clients in wheelchairs, 102
Trust, 42

V
Values, 19
concepts of, 20
defined, 20
of faculty, 21-25
framework, 25
historic, 20
professional, 20-21

Victim's Rights week, 126
Violence, in music, 44
Visiting Nurses Association (VNA), 150, 154
collaborative relationship with, 153
VNA. *See* Visiting Nurses Association

W
"Walking a fine line," 63
Web site, student stories on, 37
"What if" scenarios, 64
Wheelchairs, clients in, 102
Wellness-promotion projects, 130
Westberg, Rev. Granger, 162
Writing
evaluation of, 37
expressive, 32
grading of, 37
as process, 32
transactional, 32